There Is
Something
about
Gina

There Is Something about Gina

Flourishing with Diabetes and Celiac Disease

Gina Meagher

Something About Gina, LLC

There Is Something about Gina
Flourishing with Diabetes and Celiac Disease

Published by Something About Gina, LLC
info@somethingaboutgina.com

Book design by Kerrie Lian under contract with MacGraphics Services: www.MacGraphics.net

Photo credit: cover, pg. v — Involved Channel/Shutterstock.com

Printed in the United States of America
First Printing: February 2013

ISBN: 978-0-9886068-0-7 (paperback)
eISBN: 978-0-9886068-1-4 (e-book)
LCCN: 2012921794

The information in this book is not intended or implied to be a substitute for professional medical advice, diagnosis, or treatment. All content is for general information purposes only. The author makes no representation and assumes no responsibility for the accuracy of information contained herein. NEVER DISREGARD PROFESSIONAL MEDICAL ADVICE OR DELAY SEEKING MEDICAL TREATMENT. The author does not recommend, endorse, or make any representation about the efficacy, appropriateness, or suitability of any specific tests, products, procedures, treatments, services, opinions, health care providers or other information herein and THE AUTHOR IS NOT RESPONSIBLE NOR LIABLE FOR ANY ADVICE, COURSE OF TREATMENT, DIAGNOSIS, OR ANY OTHER INFORMATION, SERVICES, OR PRODUCTS MENTIONED HEREIN.

Stories shared are recalled to the best of the author's knowledge.

Dedicated to my husband, Jim, for his unwavering love, support, and encouragement (even in the face of my expired warranty!).

A special thanks as well to my family, whose unconditional love means more to me than they know. And to my friends, whose caring and thoughtfulness is a constant source of strength.

Thanks, also, to Jerry Payne, my editor, whose ability to get me to open up, and keep me focused, helped make the writing of this book a truly rewarding experience.

Finally, this book is further dedicated to those living with chronic conditions. Those struggling, perhaps, and looking for help in finding a better quality of life. This they can find and more; for I have come to know without a doubt that beyond just living with a chronic condition, it's possible to *flourish!*

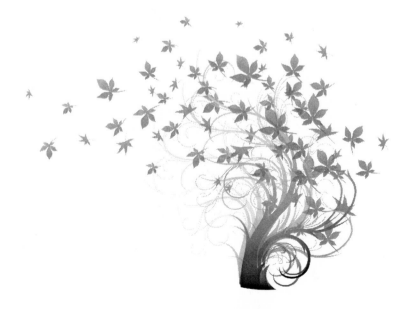

Contents

Introduction

*" It's not what happens to you,
it's what you do about it. "*

W. Mitchell

When I was seventeen, I was diagnosed with type 1 diabetes. When I was thirty-two, I was diagnosed with celiac disease (sprue). Both are chronic conditions. That means, absent the possibility of a cure, I'll have these diseases for the rest of my life.

Needless to say, such a state of affairs can be extremely challenging. It can be depressing and frustrating, inconvenient and stressful. It can be downright scary too. But in the years since my diagnoses, I've found it to be something else as well: educational. One would never wish for a chronic disease, of course, let alone two of them. But if there's a silver lining, it's this: by learning to live with my conditions, I have learned much more than just how to live with diabetes and celiac disease. I have learned a lot about life. And in the process, I have learned a lot about myself. The challenges have helped me grow as a person, perhaps more than I would otherwise have grown.

This growth has, in turn, been invaluable in my relationships with others. I have forged close friendships with people who share my conditions. I also have friendships with those who don't, but whose support and encouragement allow me to be more open about who I am. In turn, they have been more open about who they are, resulting in relationships of honesty and sharing. Together, we've learned patience and tolerance. The fact is, everyone has something to deal with. Everyone faces hardships at one time or another.

Ultimately, what I've learned is that the point isn't *what* we have to deal with; the point is how well we deal with it.

If you're living with a chronic condition or know someone who's living with a chronic condition, I believe you'll find this book of interest. But you might find it of interest as well if you're a student of life itself; if you've had your own moments of difficulty, frustration, or doubt; if you've faced your own fair share of hardships (or more than your fair share) and you're facing them still.

I won't pretend I have all the answers. What works for me might not work for you. But there are perspectives one can have — attitudes and mindsets — that can enable one to see solutions instead of problems. Those solutions might be completely specific to you and may not reflect my own experiences at all, but that's okay. I can show you where to look. I can't promise that I can solve your problems; I haven't solved mine. But what I have learned is how to *manage* them, and you can learn to manage yours too.

None of this represents ivory-tower discoveries. Nor magic, silver-bullet answers. My approach has been forged realistically over years of experience. I started out overwhelmed. The first three chapters of this book, relating my early experiences with both conditions, will certainly confirm that. But as time went on, I learned how to cope with them. I learned how to deal with societal expectations and assumptions, how to handle potential problems at the workplace, how to survive the thoughtless comments people often make, how to become empowered, how to manage my conditions, how to get the most from my doctors, and how to find support among others. I've devoted a chapter to each of these ideas. I close with some thoughts about what you can do — starting today — to make the most of your life, regardless of your challenges.

My goal is certainly not to downplay the severity of chronic disease. Those of us living with a condition as serious as diabetes realize the often frightening nature of it, the risk of debilitating complications, even death. But I learned early on that living in fear is no way to live. I knew, even then, that there had to be a better way. I hope, through this book, I can share that way with you.

For, as the title suggests, my purpose is not to suggest that you can merely live with a chronic condition. I think we can all do better than that. My purpose, as I trust you'll discover, is to suggest something more powerful. I believe — I know — that you can *flourish* with a chronic condition. My avid hope is that, by the end of this book, you'll come to believe that too.

Gina Meagher

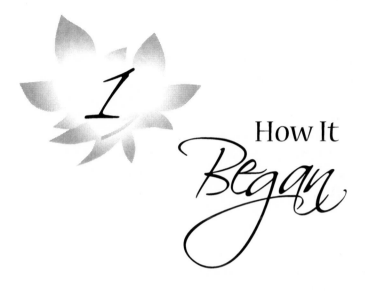

1

How It
Began

*You know what you gotta do
when life gets you down?
Just keep swimming.*

— *Finding Nemo*

"What next?" I sighed.

I'd just been given the diagnosis — the reason for my seemingly constant abdominal pain, the bloating, the diarrhea. Not to mention the fatigue. Eventually it was the anemia that had my doctor order the biopsy of my intestinal tissue, a little procedure involving a long, thin tube pushed down my throat. The biopsy had come back positive for celiac disease, an autoimmune disorder of the small intestine. (The biopsy, in fact, is the definitive test for celiac.) Individuals with celiac disease experience an immune reaction when they ingest a protein called gluten, manifesting itself in the very symptoms I had, in addition to rendering the intestine unable to absorb certain nutrients (hence the anemia). It's chronic, the doctor explained. There's no cure. I was thirty-two. And I was going to be living with celiac disease for the rest of my life.

The only treatment — eliminating gluten from one's diet — isn't as easy as it sounds. Nor is it very much fun. Gluten can be found in bread, pizza crust, pasta, beer, and basically any foods that contain wheat, barley, rye, or, to a lesser degree, oats. In time, I would learn just how many foods the list includes.

It turned out I was in a high-risk group for celiac disease because of another condition I had. Celiac disease, as it happens, wasn't my first and only chronic disease. Fifteen years earlier, at the age of seventeen, I'd been diagnosed with type 1 diabetes.

It was in October of my senior year of high school and for two or three weeks I'd been experiencing intense fatigue and an unquenchable thirst, two hallmarks of diabetes. I wasn't completely unfamiliar with the disease. Paul, a good friend, had been living with type 1 diabetes (they called it juvenile diabetes back then) since the age of twelve. Paul took shots every day, but that was about the extent of what I knew about the disease.

When I described my symptoms to him one day at school, it was like an alarm going off. "Oh, my God!" he screamed, suddenly pacing back and forth, clearly agitated. He'd seen firsthand the fatigue, the dry skin, and the weight loss, but hadn't initially pieced it together. It was the fatigue that was the most obvious indication. Reminiscing years later, he would describe "a once highly animated Gina, the life of every party, slightly hunched over, breathing deeply, almost limping through the hallway of Lindy High, a stack of text books under her arm." Even still, it wasn't until I described my severe thirst that it all came together for him, freaking him out and compelling him to insist I take a home urine test, the only real test available back in those days, outside of a doctor's office, for those with diabetes.

After school we went directly back to his house and in a little downstairs bathroom, Paul pulled out a Clinitest kit, which he used several times a day to measure his own level of glucose to better regulate the amount of insulin he'd have to inject. It involved a few drops of urine, a few drops of water, and a tablet that you combined in a little test tube. After shaking the tube, you looked at the color. If it was blue or green, you were fine. Yellow indicated a problem. Orange meant your glucose level was dangerously high. My test result was bright orange. We told Paul's mom who thought at first that maybe there was something wrong with the test. She took it herself just to see. Her test came back normal.

I went home and told my mother. She called to make an appointment to see our family doctor who insisted that, since I'd had my blood sugar tested at my last physical and it was normal, diabetes was highly improbable. That was that! No appointment made. No laboratory tests scheduled. No explanations provided. Initially I was quite relieved, but my symptoms certainly weren't going away and I knew something had to be wrong. After talking it over with Paul and some other friends a couple of days later, I decided to make an appointment for myself at a lab to have a proper test performed.

At my family physician's office, the doctor delivered the news from the lab, running a finger over my dry, swollen, chapped lips. "Yep, you have diabetes."

From there it was medication and a weeklong hospital stay. I would learn how serious the disease was, how close I'd come to dying, and how lucky it was that Paul and I persisted in getting the laboratory test. A year later I would learn it all again, going into a diabetic coma, having to be airlifted to the hospital, and having it gently suggested to my parents that, perhaps, they should begin planning their daughter's funeral. I survived — smarter, of course, but with still a lot of learning ahead of me.

Now, fifteen years later, here I was receiving another diagnosis of another chronic disease. What next?

In time, I learned how to live with celiac disease just as I'd learned to live with diabetes. In much less time, actually, since the experience of living with diabetes had provided me with a road map of sorts. I knew all about the mental stages I would go through. I knew all about the feelings of being perceived as "different." I knew I'd have to deal with ignorance masked as good intention. And I knew how emotionally dangerous it was to skirt around the bottomless "why me?" hole for too long. All of this gave me a head start towards where I knew I eventually had to be. A place where you're not controlled by the disease. A place where you're not defined by it. A place where you take charge and live your life the way that you want to. It's not always easy, and it requires a pretty serious shift in attitude. But the payoff ... the payoff is oh, so rewarding!

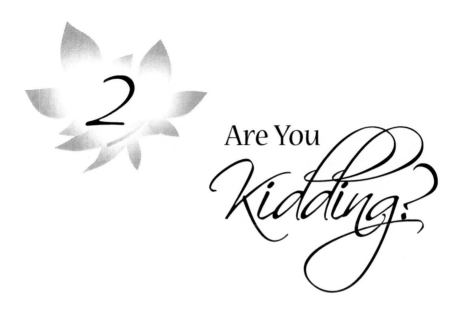

2

Are You *Kidding?*

" *Don't play the result.* "

⟶ Michael J. Fox

My weeklong hospital stay right after my diabetes diagnosis involved some basic education about the disease, including, most memorably, practicing the use of a syringe. One afternoon, a nurse in a starched, white cap placed on my dinner tray three items: a syringe, a vial of clear liquid (probably saline), and a grapefruit. I stared at her blankly.

"Okay, this is what you do," she stated matter-of-factly. I skeptically watched the step-by-step process as she demonstrated measuring out the liquid into the syringe, tapping the syringe to remove the air bubbles, and injecting the grapefruit. "There," she said. "Now you do it."

Nervously I took the syringe from her hand and repeated what I saw her do. I remember practicing this technique over and over again for a couple of days. I was apparently supposed to become comfortable with the ins and outs of how to inject myself with insulin for the rest of my life. It worked fine in theory but sticking a needle in my arm turned out to be nothing like sticking it into a grapefruit. When it's about to go into your very own skin for the first time you find yourself completely wanting to resist. Your mind rebels. You become tentative and you hesitate the same way you might hesitate if you were about to jump into a cold swimming pool. You know it isn't going to be pleasant. Every instinct tells you not to do it. Deep down, of course, I knew I needed to stick that needle into myself. And so after placing it against my arm, taking a couple deep breaths, and closing my eyes, I did it. Mainly, just to get it over with. And then I exhaled, deeply relieved. Yay! I had done it! But the feeling was short-lived. Anyone, I realized, could give themselves a shot once. But then it struck me that this was something I was going to have to go through every day for the rest of my life. What I didn't know then was how much easier it would become with time. Today I often give myself a shot while carrying on a conversation with somebody. It's almost effortless. But it sure wasn't back in those early days.

Meanwhile, the nurses and dietitians gave me some reading material about diabetes and I learned what I could about my new chronic condition. Essentially, diabetes is a metabolic disorder whereby the pancreas, an organ right under your stomach, fails to produce a sufficient quantity of insulin. The presence of insulin triggers cells to take up glucose (sugar) from the blood and store it (in the form of glycogen) for when the body needs energy. Without insulin, the cells don't do what they're supposed to do and the blood runs rampant with glucose. Bad things can result. Long-term consequences may include cardiac problems, kidney damage, limb amputation, and blindness. Short-term problems might include hyper- and hypoglycemia which can quickly lead to a coma or worse. Of course none of these things have to happen; all are preventable. But what I was learning back in those days after just being diagnosed seemed menacing, if not downright frightening.

Type 1 diabetes, which is what I was diagnosed with, means your body simply fails to produce the required insulin, whereas type 2 diabetes is a condition where your cells fail to use insulin properly. "Insulin resistance" is the term used. Type 2 is by far the more prevalent condition, accounting for about 95 percent of all diabetes cases. The primary risk factor for type 2 is being overweight, especially among those who are genetically predisposed to the disease. That means that for type 2, the disease is preventable. You can see it coming and you can take action (exercise, moderation in diet, etc.) to stop it or delay its onset. Doctors can diagnose someone as "prediabetic" and work with that individual to actually reverse the progression of the disease.

Type 1, on the other hand, is caused by your own immune system gone amiss. Instead of fighting off harmful bacteria, viruses, or parasites like it's supposed to, the system ends up attacking the very cells in the pancreas (called beta cells) that produce insulin. Nobody really knows why. Medical professionals believe there's a genetic susceptibility to type 1 diabetes, and environmental factors may play a part as well. For me, it didn't seem particularly genetic. Although my maternal grandfather was diagnosed at about the age of sixty-two, and one of my paternal aunts at eighty, both were diagnosed with type 2 diabetes. Nobody else in my family has been diagnosed, though I come from a fairly large family — four siblings, nineteen aunts and uncles, and seventy-plus first cousins. It seems likely, however, that there might be a genetic predisposition to autoimmune diseases in general, not necessarily specific ones within a family. But in any event, unlike type 2 diabetes, type 1 is not reversible. Exercise and proper diet aren't enough to get your immune system to decide to stop attacking your insulin-producing cells.

Although diabetes has been around awhile (there's mention of it in ancient Egyptian texts from about 3,500 years ago), it's only been since the 1920s that insulin has been made available for individuals to better regulate their blood sugar. Insulin is an absolute must for type 1. Type 2 can sometimes be treated with oral medication. Both types (along with a third type — gestational diabetes that occurs with some women when they become pregnant) require that you keep an eye on what you eat.

Information about the disease, when I was diagnosed, was much less available than today, and the treatment was a bit more rudimentary. I made use of basically two types of insulin, depending on how quickly I needed it to be at its maximum strength (peak) in order to properly manage my blood sugar. I had to very carefully watch what I ate, pace my eating, and try to match my insulin dosage accordingly. I remember thinking that it was all very overwhelming, and it really was, especially compared to today where there are faster-acting types of insulin and better methods of monitoring one's blood sugar. We're closer today, in other words, to being able to regulate our insulin levels the way the body does naturally — as needed over time, rather than in one fell swoop with a shot or two. It's better today, but it's still challenging.

When you're initially diagnosed, you find yourself going through the famous Kübler-Ross model of the five stages of grief: denial, anger, bargaining, depression, and, finally, acceptance. Initially, I skipped over denial. I'd been feeling deathly ill for a couple weeks prior, so much so that I couldn't even get out of bed to take my college entrance exams, which had to be rescheduled for me. My mouth was constantly dry, leading to my chapped and swollen lips. The only time I didn't feel thirsty was when I was drinking something and the liquid was actually in my mouth. I went through gallons and gallons of any type of liquid readily available and could never seem to stop feeling thirsty. Naturally I had to use the bathroom constantly. I seemed to live in the bathroom. As soon as any liquid went in, it seemed to want to come out. I lost a bit of weight too. It all added up and when the doctor confirmed my suspicions, it was hardly anything I could really deny.

At first, I spent much of my time in anger. I was seventeen years old. I had been enjoying my senior year of high school, going to parties and football games. I was researching colleges and dreaming about the future. And suddenly I was faced with a disease I would have to deal with for the rest of my life. *Why me?* I thought. *What did I do to deserve this? It was unfair. It was uncalled for. It was just plain wrong.* I was bitter and resentful.

I was also feeling buried by the amount of information that was coming at me all at once. There was a lot to learn about what I needed to do to properly handle the disease, a lot to absorb. Mostly, it seemed to me, the information, no matter how it was presented, was nothing more than just a huge laundry list of things you couldn't do — warnings about what you weren't supposed to eat, for example. Sugary food was considered off limits, obviously, what with the effects it would have on your blood sugar level. But even some of the food you could eat was listed on the pamphlets they handed me with warnings about the proper amounts. You were supposed to carefully measure everything out. "No more than seventeen small grapes," I remember reading somewhere in all the material I was bombarded with. "One small (less than six inches) banana." Since carbohydrates raise blood sugar, you had to watch the amount of carbs you consumed. "Fifteen grams of carbohydrates per serving," it said in the literature. And as an example of fifteen grams, they showed a picture of one-fourth of a standard sized bagel. At any one time I could only eat a quarter of a bagel? I remember thinking, *Who eats a quarter of a bagel?!* Collectively, all the many warnings were paralyzing.

That, I suppose, was the bargaining part of the process. Follow all the dos and don'ts and — maybe — you'll be okay. But of course, being a teenager, I didn't exactly appreciate being told what I could and couldn't do, even if it was for my own good. It wasn't a bargain I was ready for. The authoritative "Don't do this!" messages rubbed me the wrong way. But more than anything, as a teenager, you just want to be, and feel, normal. It's a time of tremendous peer pressure and nobody wants to be different. As my friend Paul put it, from his own experience with diabetes, it's okay to stand out as long as you're standing out for something great; otherwise, you just want to blend in.

I remember, shortly after I started college, sleeping in one Saturday, just a couple of hours past the time I was supposed to have gotten up to give myself a shot. Somehow it came up during a visit to the doctor's office and the doctor asked why I didn't get up when I was supposed to. I remember saying with a shrug, "Because I just wanted to feel normal." He looked up from my chart, paused for a few seconds, and nodded. And I knew by the look on his face that he got it.

It was during that first year of college when I really learned about the realities of diabetes and how quickly things can go from good to bad. We had just moved to Colorado from Long Island and I had enrolled in the University of Colorado Boulder. Somewhere I had picked up the flu and when I finished classes for the Thanksgiving break, I went home sick. Since I wasn't eating, I lowered my insulin dose. It never occurred to me that my insulin requirements would actually increase because of my illness. After a day or so of not enough insulin, my blood sugar levels rose and I passed out in the bathroom. Although I have no memory of it, I'm told my father had to break down the door. I was airlifted to the hospital where I went into a coma and my parents were told they might want to start thinking about planning my funeral.

Obviously, I recovered. Of course the experience didn't do much to help my bleak outlook. I remember a doctor at the time telling my parents, "Well, you know, it could actually be a lot worse. If you have to have a disease, diabetes isn't the worst. It's not like, say, chronic kidney disease where you're forced to undergo dialysis on a regular basis." I wasn't much interested in silver linings. I had just come out of a coma, after all. "Well, what's it matter?" I said to my mom when she repeated the doctor's sentiments to me. "I'm probably not going to live past forty-five anyway." That's the way I saw things at the time. I was depressed, frustrated, and discouraged. I thought I'd been doing okay, then just a day or so without enough insulin and I'd found myself in a coma. What was the point?

At least for the time being, however, as bleak as I thought my future was, I stopped feeling so inclined to want to rebel against the confines of the disease. You learn quickly who's in charge. In time, though, I'd also learn that while I might not be able to control diabetes, I could at least manage it. That was a major, significant change in mindset.

Managing meant, among other things, getting better at picking up cues from my body. This was difficult at first. The problem with diabetes is not just that you need insulin. It's striking the right balance between insulin, food, exercise, and the day-to-day aspects of just living. You can feel the symptoms when you're out of balance and your blood sugar is high. You feel lethargic and thirsty. So you take some insulin, but too much and you now have low blood sugar — you're shaky and weak. You need to eat something. It's a constant battle, and it wasn't always easy for me as a rookie with the condition. It's easier now, with experience, but also with the advances in monitoring and insulin therapies. Even with the advances, though, you end up listening to your body, something you just get better at with time. Still, no two days are ever alike. But over time, you learn.

For a while after being diagnosed, the frustration for me came mostly from the glucometer, that pesky device that measures your blood sugar level and tells you, in no uncertain terms, how well (or how poorly) you're managing your diabetes. I quickly developed a love/hate relationship with the glucometer. It can be your best friend and your worst enemy. It tells you what you need to know. But when you're positive you've been paying attention and eating properly and taking your insulin and doing absolutely everything right and the glucometer tells you otherwise with a reading that indicates your blood sugar level is off, you want to just take the glucometer and smash it into a million pieces. You feel like a failure. You want to give up. The glucometer becomes this ruthless and unrelenting sentry, some bizarre, unfeeling machine. But in time, I learned how to handle that too.

All of my experience with diabetes helped immensely when I ultimately learned of my diagnosis for celiac disease fifteen years later. As it turns out, there's a connection. Type 1 diabetes means you're at an increased risk for celiac disease, as well as certain other autoimmune disorders (e.g., rheumatoid arthritis and lupus).

It started with abdominal pain, often severe. It went on for months. I felt bloated, I had diarrhea. I became anemic. It was a mystery illness that my doctor originally tried to treat with a regimen of antibiotics. Eventually, the biopsy confirmed the suspicion he'd had. Strangely, I felt almost relieved. At least I knew there was a reason for my symptoms. My condition even had a name. Celiac disease, with over two-hundred potential symptoms, is not an easy disease to diagnose. Unlike type 1 diabetes, which has such obvious and specific symptoms, the symptoms of celiac disease can mimic any number of conditions, like irritable bowel syndrome, for example. For most celiacs, it can take upwards of eleven years before they ultimately get an accurate diagnosis.

With celiac disease, your small intestines have an immune reaction to the protein gluten, found in foods that contain wheat, barley, rye, or, to a lesser degree, oats. In addition to the painful symptoms, you can end up malnourished and vitamin-deficient as your small intestine becomes unable to absorb certain nutrients. The only way to manage it is to completely remove gluten from your diet. And, like diabetes, it's a chronic condition.

Once I adjusted what I ate, I felt better almost immediately. The challenge, though, would be to adjust what I ate for the rest of my life. Again, I was handed pamphlets which — again — listed all the foods that I could not eat. "Don't eat this!" "Don't eat that!" It was just as frustrating, maybe more so because now I had to factor in both sets of restrictions. *What next?* I sighed.

But the process of adapting was quicker. I was more mature. And by then I had learned a thing or two about the management of chronic conditions. I had the benefit of experience. I had already faced, and overcome, a multitude of challenges.

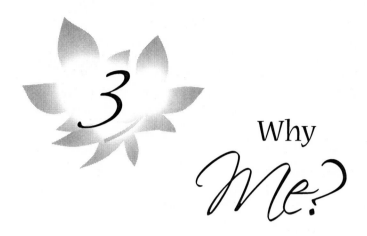

3

Why *Me?*

> " *Self-pity is our worst enemy*
> *and if we yield to it, we can*
> *never do anything wise*
> *in this world.* "
>
> Helen Keller

The lessons I learned in how to manage a chronic disease were born of necessity. With diabetes, I had to find ways to try to mentally move forward. Early on I was in danger of wallowing in self-pity and I knew deep down that if I wasn't careful, my mental state could do more damage than the disease itself.

It started with the "why me?" thoughts. It's a common response, of course, and perfectly natural. *Me? Of all the people in the world, why me?* I found myself in a state of disbelief. It was crushing and overpowering. I struggled to make some kind of sense of it, but it just seemed so random and absurd.

Strange thoughts go through your head. You wonder if there might have been something you did wrong to somehow "deserve" the disease. Maybe you're being punished in some way by a higher power. Maybe you collected a bunch of bad karma in a past life. Maybe it's the universe's way of meting out justice.

You get angry. Resentful. At the universe, at fate, at the disease, at anything and everything that you perceive played a role in your situation. The anger very slowly wears away and you're left with a sort of defeated feeling and the temptation to think of yourself as a victim. Once you attach that label to yourself, you really begin to wallow in self-pity. It becomes easy to feel sorry for yourself.

This is not to say that experiencing anger and feeling defeated are somehow out of line. They're perfectly normal and understandable reactions, even necessary as steps towards an eventual healthier outlook. Denying them only delays them. Denying them covers them up without dealing with them. You can only pretend to ignore them for so long. Sooner or later, those feelings are going to come out and so you need to find a way to handle them. I sensed this deep down, even early on. I knew that somehow I would need to find a way to deal with the negative emotions I was feeling.

And besides, the negative emotions never entirely go away. Anybody, from time to time, can become depressed dealing with a chronic condition. It's a hole that every so often you have to struggle to keep from getting sucked into.

The sense of "why me?" has a way of implying isolation and alienation. Back then I found myself looking for ways in which to prove myself "normal," as if there's any such definitive thing. As if there's some objective, unchanging standard to which everything must be compared. In truth "normal" is whatever society in general happens to find acceptable at any given point in time. But I wanted to prove myself "normal," to myself, as well as to others. I wanted to show (and feel) that I was just as "normal" as anyone, regardless of whatever condition I might have.

In high school, especially, I was very aware of how I was being perceived by others. I enjoyed going out with my friends to movies, dancing, and just hanging out. And I wasn't going to let the diabetes interfere with any of that. I made it a point not to show any type of weakness that someone might (rightly or wrongly) attribute to my diabetes. There were times at parties, for instance, when I was tired of dancing and wanted to just sit down for a while. *But how,* I wondered, *would that look?* Would people think I was tired because of the disease? Would they whisper to themselves, "Hey, there's Gina needing to rest. Think she's okay? I'll bet it's the diabetes." Sometimes, maybe it was. And yet people — "normal" people — took rests all the time, with nobody giving it a second thought. I couldn't take the chance, though. I wanted to show I was just as healthy as the next person. Maybe I wanted to prove it to myself as much as I wanted to prove it to anyone else, if not more so. The understanding of how people view us — and how we view ourselves — is, as we'll see as this book progresses, a real key to living with a chronic condition.

Of course besides the anger and depression, there's fear. Some of it is warranted. With diabetes, the complications are serious, even fatal. It's entirely appropriate to be concerned. But, left unchecked, fear can be paralyzing. Maybe it works as a motivating tool for some people, I don't know. It sure doesn't work for me. Not now, and not then. For me, the fear just made me feel stressed early on. And I knew I was eventually going to need to find a way to manage that fear. I was going to need to find some peace of mind.

There was a lot of frustration too, and not just aimed in a general way towards the disease. After a while, I could live with the idea of the disease. But there were specific moments of frustration when the disease seemed to mock my efforts at managing it. The chief offender was my glucometer — "The Machine." I would do everything I was supposed to do in order to maintain my blood sugar at the appropriate level. I would limit my grapes to the seventeen small ones that the literature recommended, or eat my small-sized banana, and live with all the other dietary recommendations, no matter how restrictive they seemed to me, then test my blood sugar and — in spite of all my conscientious efforts — the meter would tell me I failed. What?! It was infuriating. It was like studying diligently for an exam, going to the review session, pulling an all-nighter, and memorizing the text book, then confidently turning in your exam only to have it returned to you with a big red "F" scrawled across the top. *What more can I do?* I wondered. *What's the point of even trying?* I felt like a failure. All of my painstaking efforts seemed for naught.

And it was all the time. Several times a day, the unfeeling machine either provided some kind of validation or, seemingly more often than not, tagged me as a lost cause. It reminded me in no uncertain terms that I was flawed and incapable of achieving the minimum results required. Everything that was Gina was suddenly being defined by the all-powerful glucometer. What chance did I stand against it? Why go on? What's the point when the glucometer tells me I'm a failure? It's nothing less than a miracle that I didn't — even once, no matter how tempted — completely destroy the meter in a fit of frustrated rage.

It wasn't necessarily any better when the judgment was coming from a real person. Going to see the doctor periodically instilled in me additional moments of nervous apprehension. Doctor anxiety was almost as bad as the anxiety that I felt from using the glucometer. To find out how I was doing with the management of my disease seemed less like a trip to the doctor and more like a trip to the principal's office. I didn't even want to go.

I can imagine that this feeling is a big part of the reason some people living with diabetes don't, in fact, visit their doctors or go as often as they should. Later, we'll talk about how I would, eventually, make peace with the medical profession.

I was frustrated, as well, by the challenge of trying to manage my disease without altering my rather spontaneous lifestyle. I'm a person who's not afraid to act on the spur of the moment. If someone calls with an idea about doing something right now, I'm typically on board. It wasn't that hard with diabetes, at least once I got a better handle on it. At first I just tried to do what I always did, albeit with a modified diet. But there was a penalty for my sometimes erratic management. My blood sugar ended up all over the place and I wouldn't feel as well. Later on it would be easier for me with the medical advances in diabetes treatment, as well as my experience with managing my condition.

With celiac disease, it's a bit more frustrating. Many impromptu activities involve eating. "Hey, Gina, we're going out for pizza; come with us!" It can be a little awkward. It's better now than when I was first diagnosed since there are more gluten-free foods available at a wider variety of restaurants. At the time, though, it was a huge challenge, not just in restaurants, but even in shopping for foods. It was surprising to me, and depressing, to learn that gluten seemed to be in everything, seemingly hidden in foods you wouldn't even suspect would have gluten like certain soups, prepared rice mixes, or lunch meats. Sauces for seasoning are often thickened with flour. I even found out — the hard way, which is how I made many similar discoveries — that soy sauce had gluten! Wheat is the first ingredient listed.

Then of course there's accepting invitations to dinner in someone's home. You're never quite sure what you're going to get. Sometimes mashed potatoes are seasoned with spices that contain wheat. Gluten, I learned early on, appeared to be everywhere. And if you make a mistake, you might feel sick for days until the gluten works its way through your intestinal tract.

In time I found ways to handle all of the challenges that had a direct bearing on my physical well-being, and I'll share some of those ways as we move forward. But other challenges were present too, and still are. Challenges that had less to do with managing the diseases and more to do with how the people around me reacted to them.

Perceptions

The thing that is really hard, and really amazing, is giving up on being perfect and beginning the work of becoming yourself.

— Anna Quindlen

The idea of wanting to be perceived as "normal" comes in large part from the way in which society seems to view those with chronic diseases. There's a certain stigma that's attached to someone with a chronic disease — a sense that the person is weak or damaged or even defective. Somehow, you're not as "good" as people who are free of chronic conditions. It almost borders on being a judgment of character. For this reason, some people with chronic diseases become embarrassed by their conditions, almost feeling apologetic, hiding their conditions lest others find out and judge them "flawed" or "not normal." I've never felt embarrassed, exactly, but I can certainly understand the reaction, given society's point of view.

Of course the stigma is misplaced. It becomes erroneously aimed at the person and not the disease. A person with diabetes is thought of as being "a diabetic." That becomes the defining value. *Gina? Oh, yeah, she's the diabetic one.* It can make you feel as though you're walking around with a big "D" pasted on your forehead. But diabetes (or celiac disease, or any chronic condition) defines a person no more accurately than, say, the color of their hair. I am not "a diabetic" any more than I am "a brunette." Both characteristics are true, in so far as they go, but both are woefully incomplete in providing a true all-around description of Gina.

The misguided notion that you're somehow "flawed" leads people to make assumptions about what you can't do. But people living with diabetes can do most things that others can do. We may just have to plan a little bit more to take our condition into account. My husband and I are considering taking up scuba diving, for example. At one time it was considered dangerous for someone with diabetes to scuba dive. Fearful of the risk, many diving instructors wouldn't take on a student who had diabetes. But now, it's generally understood, at least by those familiar with the issue, that people with diabetes have no more real risk than anybody else. Surveys and studies have confirmed this. There are a couple caveats, of course. You need to have your blood sugar well-managed and that means you're probably going to need your doctor to sign off on any necessary medical form. So if you're like me, and you've been living with diabetes for a while and have a good handle on the management of your condition, you're fine. Naturally, you need to be in good physical shape, but isn't that the case for anyone and everyone thinking of scuba diving? After all, many of life's experiences require some level of preparation no matter who you are and no matter what conditions you may or may not have. Truthfully, my major issue with scuba diving is the idea of breathing under water! If I decide not to pursue scuba diving, it won't be because of my diabetes. If anything, it'll be because of my discomfort with the thought of getting my air out of a cylindrical, metal tank.

As a person living with diabetes, I believe I can do anything I put my mind to. I suppose I've always felt this way, and diabetes hasn't done anything to dispel the idea. I'm the shortest of four girls and as kids we all played basketball. I still do. But I knew I couldn't compete with my sisters right under the basket. With two or four inches on me, they had the advantage. But I wanted to play, and I wanted to be good. So I adapted. I worked on becoming a guard, shooting from the perimeter and playing tough defense. Quick and scrappy, my sisters described me. I found, in other words, a way in which to adapt so that I could do what it was I wanted to do and not embarrass myself in the process.

It's an idea that I've carried with me throughout the trials and tribulations of both my chronic conditions. If I really want to do something, I'll find a way to do it. It becomes my choice. I don't allow the diseases to dictate what I can and cannot do any more than I allowed my lack of relative height to dictate whether or not I could enjoy basketball.

It's an attitude that those around me are intimately familiar with. I have a now-grown niece, Sarah, who remembers fondly growing up and spending time with Aunt Gina. She would ask about my diabetes, always very curious about the shots and my management of the disease. For her, it just became second nature. Though it might have been a curiosity, it wasn't an issue and never a problem. As she remembers it, "We had better things to worry about, like figuring out how many water parks and mini-golf games we could fit into one day. We kids always knew that Aunt Gina was going to have fun no matter what."

What's unfortunate about allowing yourself to be stopped by the disease is that that actually feeds into the societal view that there are things you cannot do. The misperception grows. I must admit I end up losing patience with those who allow that to happen, even though I realize it's due to a certain level of fear. If the fear is warranted, of course it's understandable that someone would be reluctant to try something. But many times the disease is simply used as an excuse. The key is to be honest with yourself. If you really feel as though you want to challenge yourself with scuba diving, rock climbing, hang gliding, or whatever, but find yourself hesitating, ask yourself if it's really the disease, or if you're using the disease as an excuse.

For me, doing what I really want to do might just mean preparing a little differently than someone else who might not have diabetes. Maybe my preparation might necessitate an extra step or two. And a lot of the preparation for me comes about as a result of experience — knowing how my body reacts and adjusting accordingly. Over the years I've learned how to listen to what my body is telling me. I know, for example, that when I intensely play racquetball for an hour, my blood sugar is going to rise a little. But I also know that in about two to four hours, it'll return to normal. Consequently, I resist the temptation to take additional insulin right away. I also know that when I spend a couple hours on the golf course, my blood sugar is going to dip. Typically, then, I'll reduce my insulin by one or two units prior to playing and bring a little something along to eat in case I need it. These were approaches that I had to learn over time. And they're tailored, of course, to my particular needs. Other people may react differently. The point is, if you can learn to pay attention to the signs your body is giving you, you can properly prepare.

In addition to making assumptions about what you can and can't do, people often make assumptions about how you got the disease in the first place. I imagine this is true with a lot of chronic conditions but it seems to be especially true with diabetes. There's a societal perception that diabetes means being overweight or obese, and being overweight or obese, of course, has its own stigma and set of misconceptions. If you're obese, so society thinks, you lack self-control and are too lazy to work out. It's terribly unfair, of course. It's unfair to people who are overweight, those with type 2 diabetes (which does indeed come with a risk factor having to do with being overweight, although it's only one of several), and even more unfair for those with type 1 diabetes, which doesn't typically come with such a risk factor. And yet, that doesn't stop people from telling me, since I'm not obese or overweight, "Really? You don't look like you have diabetes!" In the early days of my disease, I was known to sometimes testily answer, "Really? What *should* I look like?" Fortunately, I've matured and have decided to take it as the compliment it's probably meant as. "Thanks," I'll say, and leave it at that.

Most of the problems regarding society's viewpoint of people with chronic conditions come from a place of relative ignorance. People just simply don't know. This might explain why many people are uncomfortable talking to someone with diabetes, or any chronic condition, about their disease. When I tell people I live with diabetes, sometimes they'll simply clam up. "Oh," they'll say. They'll try to give me an understanding look, and then they'll start searching for another topic of conversation. They may be afraid of saying the wrong thing, or they may just feel as though they have nothing to add. If they don't know enough about diabetes, because they have no firsthand experience with diabetes, they might feel they have nothing to offer. They may feel as if they're not qualified to say anything. Yet, if someone came to me saying they were getting divorced, I might feel inclined to offer a word or two of support, even though I have no firsthand experience with divorce. Problems of the human condition — illness, divorce, death of a loved one, loss of one's job — these are all universal problems. We all have some experience with the struggles and emotions of other people because we've all experienced struggles and emotions in our own lives, even if the particulars were different. And if nothing else, a person can still just be there as a sounding board.

The fact is, most people would be surprised at how open-minded I can be to someone's suggestions or ideas, so long — and this is important —so long as the input comes from a sincere and a nonjudgmental position. If someone is trying to be helpful and asking sincere questions about my condition(s), then I become interested in what they have to say about it. You just never know what someone with a completely different perspective can offer.

Whether or not to share with others the particulars of your chronic condition, or even that you have a chronic condition, is a personal choice. It's one that everybody has to decide for themselves. There are situations where you may have to disclose your disease — in the workplace, for instance, or maybe on an application for scuba-diving instruction. With other situations, such as social situations with acquaintances and friends, you have options. It's common for people to wonder just whom they should tell and when. How best to decide just might depend on the type of person you are.

In her research of the brain, Dr. Geil Browning of Emergenetics International (www.emergenetics.com) discovered that people have different behavioral and thinking preferences.

Maybe you will recognize your preferences in the descriptions below. Recognizing your preferences might help you determine how to go about letting (or not letting) people know about your condition or conditions.

Behavior attributes are what people may see in you, how they would describe you. Dr. Browning identified three *behavioral* preferences — expressiveness, assertiveness, and flexibility.

Your degree of **expressiveness** indicates the amount of your social participation with others. It's not what you experience inwardly, but what you share outwardly. Your degree of expressiveness may determine how much of your condition you wish to share with others. If you are an introverted or reserved person, you may have a difficult time opening up about your chronic condition(s) to others. You may choose to discuss your condition with as few people as possible. If, however, your degree of expressiveness indicates that you are extroverted and outgoing, you may want to tell everyone you meet. In that case, open communication might be best for you. Tell your friends; tell *all* your friends. Let them support you, lift you up, and feed energy back to you. You'll feel better knowing your friends know about your disease, and knowing that you have nothing to hide from them. It may also help you come to terms with your condition(s).

The next behavior preference is **assertiveness**. Our degree of assertiveness reflects the amount of energy we invest in expressing our thoughts, feelings, and beliefs. Your degree of assertiveness will clearly influence how you approach your condition and how you will engage with and discuss it with others. If you are a peacekeeper, someone who is easygoing and who learns by listening, you may not want to put a lot of energy into sharing what you are going through or how you are feeling. Or you may be an individual who is on the other end of the spectrum and is competitive or driven and more likely to want to

27

inform others. With this inclination you're likely to handle the uncertainties of the disease relatively well and will take charge and be very direct when communicating with others.

Finally, let's address our degree of **flexibility**. Flexibility reveals how we accommodate the thoughts and actions of others. Depending on your degree of flexibility, you may need time to adapt to the disease and how it will impact your life. The early uncertainly of the disease and what it will mean to you may be challenging. You may prefer to learn in defined situations and can be accused of being stubborn and inflexible. For you, once you begin to understand the disease and build your plan for managing it, you will be extremely focused and will cope well with a specific plan. If you are on the other end of the spectrum, you will deal well with the early ambiguity of the disease and are likely to be very open to the suggestions and ideas of others. You may enjoy getting a variety of input from all types of different people. You will need, however, to be careful about focusing and deciding on your course of action and not allowing yourself to get too distracted from your plan.

For my part, personality testing has revealed that I'm right smack in the middle on these preferences. For me, my behavior seems to be situational-based. On some things, I can be flexible and let go. On other things, I dig my heels in and become stubborn and unmoving. It all depends on what's at stake. This turns out to be perfectly consistent with how I approach others when it comes to talking about my chronic conditions. I regard each person — each situation — differently. For me, it depends on the larger picture — what my overall goal is.

And that brings us to Dr. Browning's four *thinking* preferences — analytical, structural, social, and conceptual. If your thinking preference is **analytical**, then you are likely going to want to fully research and understand your disease and how it is going to impact you. You'll approach the research in a logical way and persevere until all your questions are answered. For you the more data the better! Analyzing the data is fun; like putting a puzzle together. The challenge for you might be how you share what you are experiencing with others. Remember that you're in control. You can share in a way that reflects who you are; perhaps by sharing the data, your analysis, your findings, it might make it easier for you to discuss your disease.

If you're thinking preference is **structural**, then you will want to approach your disease in the most practical way. You likely prefer to know all the details and have a practical step-by-step approach in dealing with the changes in your routine. Though at first you may be challenged by the change in your routine, once you have a planned approach you will likely have an easier time *dealing with the structure now needed in your routine.* For diabetes, especially, you'll have a leg up on knowing how to structure your day, when to check your blood sugar levels, what you've eaten, etc. It'll all come more naturally to you. You may take a more structured approach to sharing; identifying, for example, who needs to know or who would want to know. You can even work out a schedule and system to reach out to others on your terms.

If your thinking preference is **social**, then the key question you will have is, "how do I feel about this disease?" Your reaction will be all about your feelings. You have a natural preference for connecting with other people and may even find yourself worrying about upsetting people by telling them. Your reaction to your disease may be emotional, but your intuition will mean that you will know instinctively what to share with other people and who to share it with. You will likely gain energy from sharing and interacting with the people you identify as needing to know. Being able to discuss your disease with people you trust or with other people who have experience with the disease will be important for you.

If you are like me and you prefer to see the bigger picture then you are likely a **conceptual** thinker. You have a natural ability to deal with change and are open to new concepts. You also see situations from different vantage points, so you may be able to adapt to the change quickly and bring your own unique perspective and experimental approach to dealing with it. You do not like to get bogged down in the day-to-day details. You probably don't like lists. Or, you might find them useful — for you, it depends entirely on the context. You may find that telling people what is going on is conceptually easy for you, but their responses might be difficult to manage. Some people might ask all sorts of detailed questions about blood sugar, timing, shots, foods you can eat, foods you can't eat, etc. This might drive you nuts if it comes all at once. It's best to set parameters right up front. You may start with, "I'm going to share something with you," then maybe let them know that you may not want to get into more specific details just then but maybe at a later time.

In reality, most of us are a combination of more than one thinking preference and each of our behavioral preferences are by degrees. The important takeaway is for you to recognize your preferences and then plan your response or course of action based on who you are. When we can act within our preferences, it gives us energy, so be good to yourself!

Regardless of your personality type, your preferences for opening up to others and sharing may change and evolve over time. What may unfortunately not change are the perceptions of society in general. But know that those who really love you won't label you. They'll know the disease is just something you happen to be living with and not who you are.

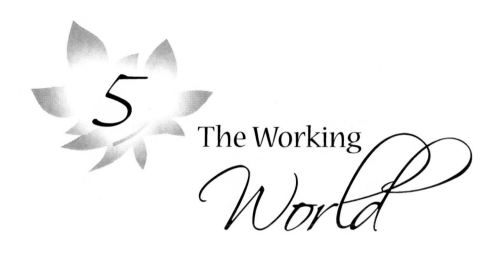

5

The Working World

" *Always bear in mind that your own resolution to succeed is more important than any other.* "

—Abraham Lincoln

In the previous chapter, we talked about dealing with others. And having to deal with friends and family is one thing. But the workplace presents its own set of challenges. Who do you tell? Who, ethically and legally, needs to know about your condition? How can you make sure your condition doesn't affect your work performance or adversely affect your interactions with others?

For my part, I'm quite comfortable with the idea that I can handle the responsibilities of my corporate job with no problems stemming from either of my conditions. My celiac disease is essentially a nonfactor, coming into play perhaps only when the issue of where to go to lunch comes up. When it comes to my diabetes, probably only a handful of the people I have ever worked with knew I was living with it. I will always tell my boss and I might tell other company personnel if I feel they should know. I traveled on business to Mexico one time with a few of my colleagues and I made sure that at least one person in the traveling party knew about my diabetes, just in case of an emergency. If nothing else, I thought it was just common courtesy to give them a heads-up.

Other people may learn about it if it happens, for whatever reason, to come up in conversation and I decide to share with them that I am a person living with diabetes. In that case, however, it would probably be part of a dialogue that's more in the way of a social, rather than work-related, interaction, and so I'd use roughly the same guidelines as in the previous chapter in deciding whether or not to tell. If, in other words, you're deciding whom to tell in the workplace about your chronic condition (outside of those who, for whatever reason, really need to know), it might depend on your personality. Are you more open with your thoughts and more comfortable letting others know, or are you more reserved and more comfortable keeping things closer to the vest? Remember that, no matter how friendly and gregarious your colleagues are, friends at work are different than other friends. You might want to err on the side of caution and if there's no particular reason for a coworker to know of your chronic condition, you may want to refrain from telling them.

I found this out one time when several fellow employees filed a well-deserved complaint about another employee — a coworker who was something of a bully. The company's human resources department did an investigation, which confirmed the account of the person's actions. They interviewed several employees in the process, including me since the coworker in question was one I often had to interact with. Apparently one of the people interviewed suggested that the bullying tactics might have bothered me more because of my diabetes. It was an ignorant comment, suggested as an apparent attempt to explain away the bullying behavior as mere oversensitivity on my part. As it turned out, I didn't have much time to be concerned about it. The director of the organization found out about the comment and, furious that someone would make an issue of my condition, gave the other employee an earful. The bottom line is, having to hear thoughtless comments is one reason why I prefer to keep the people I work with on a need-to-know basis.

When looking for a job or being interviewed for one, I rarely feel the need to bring up my diabetes right away. I consider the requirements of the job and make a determination as to whether my condition might in any way affect my job performance, or if for some odd reason my condition might put me or those around me at risk (in which case I'd beg off, though I have yet to come across such a position). If job performance is the issue, I look for ways in which my condition might need to be accommodated. If I'm directly asked during the interview process if there's anything about me that might interfere with my duties, I'm honest. All in all, however, it's hard for me to imagine a job I could not do if I really wanted to. And I have been fortunate in my experience; no potential employer, that I know of, has considered my condition to be a reason not to hire me.

In fact, the closest I've come to witnessing potential discrimination actually happened to someone else. A coworker with type 1 diabetes was having an especially hard time managing it. The company, to its credit, made appropriate allowances for him, even allowing him to work odd shifts and hours. But I sensed an underlying current of resentment from the other employees, even though in some ways they were benefitting from the allowances made to him. Some of the employees made comments to me — unaware that I, too, live with diabetes — insinuating that if the employee in question can't do his job the way everybody else has to do theirs, he should be let go. They implied that he was getting "preferential treatment." Of course they didn't know the full story because our employer was prohibited by HIPAA regulations (**The Health Insurance Portability and Accountability Act of 1996**) from disclosing the man's condition or why they made the allowances they made. But the truth was, he was doing his job and doing it well. Had he not been, I would not have hesitated to recommend an alternative course of action. The company was doing the right thing by accommodating him. After all, they weren't doing anything more than what one would hope they'd do for every other employee, with or without a chronic condition.

On the other hand, any employee with a chronic condition needs to take individual responsibility for reducing the likelihood that his or her condition will affect his or her job performance any more than absolutely necessary. Right or wrong, a perception from other employees that you're getting preferential treatment will always breed some level of resentment. If you want to be treated like everyone else, you can't demand, or even expect, anything more than reasonable efforts to accommodate your specific needs. A chronic condition must never be used as an excuse to get preferential treatment or as an excuse for nonperformance.

My own efforts at managing my diabetes keep the need for special accommodations to a minimum. I do my best to seek ways to work around my condition as best I can. During my tenure at one particular company, I happened to be taking a type of insulin that peaked around lunchtime. Consequently, I was careful not to schedule any meetings around that time of day. Nobody ever noticed. Years later, I was talking to my supervisor from those days and somehow this came up in conversation. It surprised her. "Didn't you ever wonder why I rarely scheduled meetings for around lunch?" I said. She had to think for a moment. "Now that you mention it …" she said. But of course it was never an issue. Her next comment was especially interesting: "So, in other words, Gina, you've found ways to *manage* your diabetes so that it doesn't affect what you do?" "Exactly!" I said. And of course knowing me the way she did, she also knew that my management meant that my diabetes never had a negative effect on those around me either.

Of course that's the key. Management. Where your chronic condition is concerned, the workplace isn't any different than the rest of your life. You take action. You adapt. You adjust. You figure out work-arounds. As my former supervisor perceptively noted, you manage.

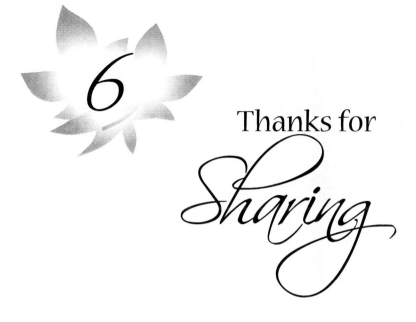

6

Thanks for *Sharing*

> " *Be kind whenever possible.*
> *It is always possible.* "
>
> — Dalai Lama

At a party recently, the movie *The Sound of Music* came up in conversation. I don't really remember how, but it seems to come up in conversation about once a year, or whenever the movie gets shown on television. I like the film. Sure, it's a little sappy, but it's a true story about a very serious time (World War II). I always cringe a little when people start talking about it because, sure enough, just like at this party, someone's going to say what this particular party guest, commenting on the overall sweetness of the movie, said: "That movie would put a diabetic into a coma!"

Funny? Well, no, not really. Especially if you're a person living with diabetes or know someone who is. In this person's defense, she had no idea I was living with diabetes. It wasn't meant to be a hurtful comment in any way. I knew she was only trying (unsuccessfully) to be funny. Those at the party who knew of my condition glanced over at me, I suppose to see my reaction or maybe in anticipation of what I was going to say. But I said nothing and as best I can recall, someone else started talking about Julie Andrews and the moment passed. Besides, I'm not the type to get on a soapbox and preach; that's just not my style. When the timing is right, I prefer to educate rather than lecture.

The truth of the matter is that if you have a chronic condition, you're going to face your fair share of uninformed, often insensitive remarks that make light (or even fun) of your condition. Some come out of the blue, like *The Sound of Music* comment, where the person making the remark simply didn't know there was a person living with diabetes in the room (and apparently never stopped to even consider the possibility). Other remarks, meanwhile, are, perhaps, well-intentioned and spoken because the person knows you're living with diabetes, or maybe just found out, and feels compelled to say something.

This is where you'll find society's viewpoint, as discussed in chapter four, brought down to the individual level. People who feel obligated to say something often bring their preconceived (often societal) views with them. "You don't look like you have diabetes" is the perfect example. It's completely natural to feel as if you need to comment on something when it's brought to your attention. If it somehow comes out in conversation that I am a person living with diabetes, or celiac, or both, I have to expect that. Although some people might say nothing or attempt to change the subject, most will feel as though they have to say something. They may actually feel uncomfortable not saying something.

In this case, the question is, what should be said? Maybe the best approach is for you to guide the conversation, thus relieving the other person from having to grope around for something to say. Maybe what ends up being said is said by you. And of course what that might be will depend on the context of the conversation. How exactly did it come up? Try to allow the conversation to flow naturally towards why the information was shared in the first place, giving the other person the opportunity to respond, hopefully appropriately.

People will still, unintentionally or carelessly, make insensitive comments from time to time. I've had people say, "Wow, I could never handle giving myself shots! How many do you take?" In fact, I seem to remember saying the exact same thing to my friend Paul back in high school before I was diagnosed. But I happen to know firsthand that if you have to take shots in order to live, you take shots. It's a simple, black-and-white choice. Paul put it to me like this: "Gina, you gotta do what you gotta do." People mean no harm, of course, by remarking about how they could never take the shots. Typically, they're trying to be encouraging. It's a way of saying, "Wow, aren't you incredibly brave for being able to give yourself shots all the time!"

Sometimes, as in the case of my five-year-old niece, Amy, remarks about taking shots are made simply out of curiosity.

"What would happen, Aunt Gina," she asked one morning at the breakfast table, "if you didn't take your shots?"

"Well," I replied, without even thinking, "I would die."

Maybe I should have sugarcoated my response or found a better way to answer the question. But Amy seemed genuine with her question and so my natural reaction was to give her a truthful answer. Apparently it was a satisfactory one because she said, "Oh. Okay," and we went right on with eating our breakfast.

I've also had people say, "Well, diabetes is a lot easier to deal with these days, isn't it? Just give yourself a shot and you're good to go!" That one reminds me of what the doctor said to my parents after I'd been hospitalized: "As far as diseases are concerned, diabetes isn't the worst." Both comments are meant to be somehow cheerful, but both end up sort of trivializing your condition. It's not a big deal, is the underlying message. Well, it really is a big deal, with real consequences.

Some people want to sympathize and find a way to relate to your condition and to find a little common ground. "You know, I had an uncle with diabetes." That's fine as far as it goes. But then others feel compelled to follow that up with, "He lost his leg to the disease." Needless to say, I don't find that kind of statement very helpful or encouraging. The comment typically produces an awkward silence (what am I supposed to say?) and then the person normally jumps in with a remark designed to bail us both out of the moment. Something along the lines of, "That won't happen to you, though, Gina. I can see that you take good care of yourself. My uncle didn't."

Some comments are overly presumptuous, such as "Should you be eating that?" It makes you think the person saying it is, in a roundabout way, telling you how to live your life. The exasperated, irritated reaction would be, "Seriously? You're telling *me*, someone who's had to live with diabetes for three decades, what to eat? Really?"

My reactions have been as varied as my moods. In my best moments, I try to remember that whatever is being said is being said with the best of intentions. I either let the offending remark slide or maybe I use it as a teaching moment. "Well, actually," I might say, "I can eat this as long as I compensate for it." In my worst moments, well, there's always the impatient, irritated response. Fortunately, those moments are fewer and farther between than when I was first diagnosed. Living with my conditions over time has taught me patience, and given me a little thicker skin. But I'm not perfect; I still think about responding with statements that I'm sure I will later regret. Like the management of my diabetes, patience is apparently a day-to-day affair.

Sometimes, like with my niece, Amy, people are just curious and like to ask a lot of questions. I'm fine with this as long as I know the questions are sincere, and most of the time they are. I consider it a good opportunity to educate and inform. And it's nice to know that the other person cares enough to ask.

The truly hurtful things are often the things that are left unsaid. Like at a dinner party when someone is passing around dessert and offers everyone in the room a piece of cake but you. When that happens to me, I know the host or hostess is just trying to be sensitive to my diabetes and trying to be helpful in their own way by not putting something tempting within my grasp. But it's always awkward at best and exclusionary at worst. It makes me feel isolated. It singles me out and I feel different from everybody else. Everyone else is offered a choice of whether or not to accept the dessert. Why shouldn't I be given the same choice? "Cake, Gina?" "No, but thank you." That's all it would take.

Or — who knows? — I might want to enjoy the cake. Maybe I'd planned for it in my managing efforts. I'm the one who knows best how to manage my diabetes and what I should or should not be eating and when. When a host or hostess makes a conscious decision not to offer me dessert, I feel as though he or she is undermining how I manage my condition. It's almost an unspoken way of saying, "Should you be eating that?"

At least that's the way I see it. I know of other people living with diabetes, and/or celiac disease, who would consider it offensive, even hurtful and insensitive, to be offered something their host or hostess knows they shouldn't have. They think of it in the same way that you might think of offering an alcoholic a drink — something you should just never do. I know this makes it challenging for a host or hostess, not knowing exactly which way to proceed, so I would only suggest perhaps a middle ground. If you're unsure what your guest's preference is, how about something generic and neutral? "We're having dessert," you might say. "Can I get you anything?" Or, "Please help yourself." The key is to find a way to include everybody.

Feeling excluded is even worse when it happens on a larger scale. I've been bypassed when it comes to entire meals and entire evenings out. Because of my celiac disease, people may feel awkward about asking me out to a restaurant that they suspect may not have appropriate food options for me. And so if it happens that a group of friends is getting together at such a restaurant, I might not even be asked to come along. Talk about feeling excluded.

What's forgotten is that getting together at a restaurant is about much more than sitting down at the same table to eat some food. It's about finding an opportunity to be around your friends, to socialize, to converse, to find and share common interests, and to enjoy each other's company. It's disappointing when you find out after the fact that such an opportunity was withheld from you because, "Well, Gina, we figured you wouldn't be able to eat anything there and so we just assumed you wouldn't want to go." Like the cake example, you'd at least like to be given the option.

And just in case sparing one's feelings isn't enough of a reason to invite the person along, there are other reasons to do so. It might be that the person can work around the perceived problem. Many restaurants these days — ones run by business-savvy people — have gluten-free foods on the menu to accommodate those who are living the gluten-free lifestyle. Menu items are often marked "G.F." for Gluten-Free. My family and friends all know this. For us, G.F. stands for "Gina-Friendly" and it's our way of acknowledging my condition. When I use the phrase "Gina-Friendly," people usually smile and often take it as a personal challenge to seek out G.F. options. "Gina-Friendly" sounds a lot less intimidating than "Gluten-Free." It adds just a bit of levity. For restaurants that don't have Gina-Friendly foods, I can always just pack something in my bag. Keep in mind that it's not always about the food. I'm there for the atmosphere, the social interaction, and the camaraderie.

On rare occasions, however, I'm aware that the evening out may actually be about the restaurant. Maybe a new place has opened up and everyone wants to try it. Hopefully it's run by business-savvy people and has Gina-Friendly food, but what if it doesn't? Like the cake example, I'd still like to be offered the choice. "Gina, we're all going to that new place out by the mall on Friday. Want to come with us?" Now I have options. I can call the new place and see what their G.F. choices look like or maybe bring something of my own. Many restaurants don't mind this once the reason for doing so is explained to them.

Still, even with these available solutions, some people might not ask me along because they would think it impolite to eat foods in front of me that I cannot eat. It's not. What's impolite is not being asked to come along. If the restaurant doesn't have G.F. foods, if for some reason I don't want to pack something of my own to eat, or if I really don't want to be in a place where there's nothing but un-Gina-Friendly foods around, I can always say, "Not this time, but thanks for asking."

The comments that are said and those that are left unsaid are always going to be lurking around. There can be no stopping them. You can slow their advance by educating those around you — your friends and family and coworkers — but people are still going to inadvertently say (or leave unsaid) insensitive or hurtful comments. You can only control how you react to them.

Someone once asked me how I'd respond to having someone tell me he or she had diabetes and I didn't even have to guess. I have, in fact, had people — people who didn't know of my condition — tell me they had diabetes. Typically I would nod understandingly and respond appropriately for the context, offering support or encouragement, maybe asking a probing question or two. Doing that helps me determine how interested they are in talking about it, or how far to take the conversation. Maybe they're just looking for a sympathetic ear to vent their frustrations, their fears, or their challenges. Again, a lot depends on how the topic came up in the first place. If it was appropriate for the situation, I might mention my own diabetes. But not always. First of all the conversation isn't about me, it's about the other person. Secondly, although diabetes and celiac disease are part of who I am, they have little to do with what I am about. By understanding this, a person living with a chronic condition can begin the process of empowerment.

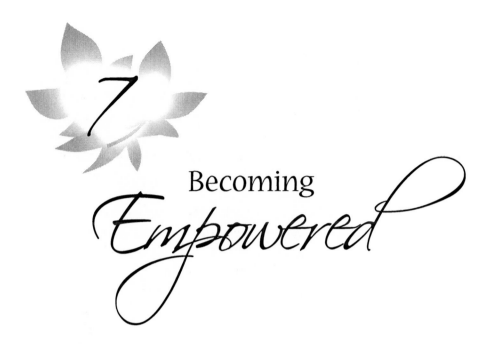

7

Becoming
Empowered

> " *If you don't like something, change it.*
> *If you can't change it, change your attitude.* "
> —Maya Angelou

Here are just a few details, some more interesting than others, about your humble author: I have brown hair. I wear glasses. I like to travel, particularly to Ireland, the country of my birth and ancestry. I'm married. I grew up on Long Island and still get teased about my New York accent. I live in Colorado. I like to sample different wines, particularly dry white wines. I enjoy sports, both as a participant and spectator. I value spending time with family and friends.

Oh, and I live with diabetes. And I also live with celiac disease.

Why didn't I mention those last two things first? Because in any attempt to summarize who I am by listing some of my characteristics, those two aspects typically don't even come to mind. As I mentioned in the last chapter, diabetes does not define me, nor does celiac disease. They are two attributes about me out of hundreds. Nothing more.

This is why, when I share that I live with diabetes, I put it into those words. I live with diabetes. Notice I don't say that "I'm a diabetic." Once you fall into the trap of referring to yourself as a diabetic, then you're allowing yourself, however unintentionally, to be defined by the disease. This may seem a minor point. It's just semantics, right? Well, the manner in which you describe yourself sticks with you. Hearing it said that you're a diabetic, or thinking of yourself as a diabetic, will, over time, bore itself into your very psyche. You'll become a diabetic, meaning that your condition becomes your prevailing characteristic, the way in which you define yourself.

Some words in particular have especially negative connotations. I've heard it said, for example, that if I eat something I'm not "supposed" to eat then I'm "cheating" on my diet. What do we call someone who's cheating? A cheat! A cheat is certainly not a name I want to be associated with, nor how I even remotely think of myself.

From where exactly does this idea of what I'm "supposed" to be eating even come? We get it into our heads that there's some objective one-size-fits-all standard that works for all situations, or for all individuals. But once you come to understand that there are no such one-size-fits-all standards, then you come to realize that the choices you make about your diet (or anything you do, for that matter) are really up to you.

When I first discovered this, it was tremendously empowering. I began to realize that I had choices I could make. If I wanted a piece of cake, I could have one as long as I properly compensated for it by adjusting my insulin intake accordingly. It wasn't cheating, and I was not a cheat. The funny thing is that early on I discovered, oftentimes, that a small taste of the cake was enough for me. Telling me I couldn't or shouldn't eat it was what made me want it so much in the first place. It's human nature. Once I made the decision that I could have it, much of the desire went away. In other words, it wasn't the cake. It was the *freedom to choose*. That was the important distinction.

I came to feel this same way regarding my celiac disease. I know that if I eat gluten now, the effects are extremely uncomfortable and might even cause me long-term problems. Consequently, I choose not to eat foods with gluten. I could eat them, mind you. I choose not to. And therein lies a powerful difference. It's the difference between the disease telling you what to eat and what not to eat, and you making up your own mind as to what to eat and what not to eat. It's a whole different perspective. There is no "supposed to" and there is no "cheating." There are simply choices.

The cheating idea arrived on the scene for me during those early years when I was seemingly fighting the glucometer at every turn. It was accusatory, that meter — that Machine. If it showed that my blood sugar was not at the appropriate level, then it was as if it was pointing a finger and calling me a cheater. Worse than accusing me of cheating, it made me feel like a failure. It was discouraging and depressing. In many ways, it actually became a deterrent in my efforts to properly manage my condition. I didn't want to even deal with The Machine.

In retrospect, I think my reaction to The Machine was rooted in fear. A bad reading was threatening. The disease suddenly became very real to me and I was rudely reminded of the potential complications. Any thoughts of denial I might have been harboring were abruptly dispelled and I would react in anger and frustration. All I knew at the time, though, was that I hated The Machine.

But somewhere along the line I began fighting back. I decided that no device was going to label me a cheater and/ or failure. I was always going to try my very best to manage my blood sugar and that was that. That's all you can really do. All you can do is your best. I used the glucometer readings as guides and made adjustments as necessary. That's all the readings ultimately became for me. Nothing more. They were representative of single points in time, revealing patterns perhaps, or trends that I needed to watch carefully.

Sometimes my adjustments were dead on. Sometimes, however, they weren't. But that became okay. I began to give myself permission to fail. It wouldn't be the end of the world if my blood sugar — at one single point in time — wasn't where it was supposed to be. I would take note of it, check the next reading, look for a pattern, think back to what I might have eaten or what activity I might have been engaged in, and, armed with this information, make an appropriate adjustment.

It's a process, in other words. An ongoing one that continues to this day. Naturally, I might have to deal with some readings with more of a sense of urgency; if my blood sugar is really high or really low, I'll have to make an adjustment right there and then. But I'll still make a note to see if it's part of some larger pattern. And because it's an ongoing process, there really isn't a stopping-off place where you "arrive." Sometimes I'm right where I want to be, but sometimes I'm not. When I'm not, that's okay. Every day the process starts anew. It's like life itself: a journey, rather than a destination.

The process has taught me patience. Sometimes (oftentimes) the successful management of a chronic condition is done by baby steps. When you're not where you want to be it's easy to get frustrated and discouraged. With patience and a long-term outlook, however, a lot of the frustration and discouragement goes away.

At times I think in terms of worst-case scenarios. What's the worst case if I eat a piece of candy? I'm unlikely to go blind right on the spot or go into an immediate diabetic coma. One piece of candy, one bad glucometer reading — these things aren't going to kill me. Lots of candy over time might kill me. But with the potential for putting on weight and hypertension and cardiovascular disease, isn't that the case for everybody? In other words, we all have to make choices. That's just the trade-off for maintaining good health, diabetes or no diabetes.

Along with patience, I've also learned tolerance. The fact of the matter is that everyone has something to deal with. Sometimes it's obvious — a person in a wheelchair, for example. But most times it's not — a person with diabetes or celiac, a person going through a divorce, a person who just lost their job, a person fighting depression. We meet people every day or pass them on the street and we imagine them to be living smooth, carefree lives. But a lot of people don't live such lives, at least not all the time. Who knows what problems are consuming another person's thoughts? I've learned, because of my own conditions, to try to take that into account when I meet someone, especially before judging him or her.

It's another reason to dispense with the "why me?" thoughts. Life isn't fair. You may as well ask why not you. Things happen. Our lives change. But life goes on. Surrendering to victimhood doesn't help. It's a perfectly understandable perspective and one I wallowed in at first. Eventually, though, you come to understand that life is going to go on, chronic condition or no chronic condition, and you have to grab a hold of it before too much of it goes by without you.

None of this happens overnight. Changing your perspective, changing your attitude, developing patience, empowering yourself, it all takes time. It took me years. But I've given my-self permission to fail on this score as well. Having a chronic condition can simply be downright depressing at times. There are days when I find myself feeling low and melancholy. But if I don't always have a positive attitude about my conditions, if I find myself sometimes wallowing just a bit, that's okay. I know I'll feel better tomorrow. What I've learned is that managing the conditions means managing my emotional outlook about the conditions too.

Since I've given myself permission to fail, I've also given myself permission to celebrate my successes. When I take a reading, for instance, and it's confirmed that what I've been do-ing is working, I do the "Snoopy dance," and if you've watched Charlie Brown specials, you know exactly what that means. Nothing celebrates success better than a good Snoopy dance. If dancing isn't your style, then find your own way to celebrate. Shout out, "YES!" Give yourself a high-five! Fist pump! Do something! The point is to find a way to cheer yourself on for your accomplishments. You deserve it.

It's important to understand that putting your disease into its proper perspective doesn't mean taking it lightly. Yes, you have choices. But it should go without saying that your choices need to be intelligent ones. Sometimes, even with your best ef-forts, diabetes (or celiac or any chronic condition) is going to be difficult to get a handle on. There's a big difference between viewing your situation (a bad glucometer reading, for instance) as a temporary setback or panicking about it (or feeling like a failure). That panic (or feeling of failure), left to its own devices will lead to another sort of chronic condition — one of con-stant fear and anxiety. Feelings of wanting to give up begin to take over all aspects of your everyday life.

It's a feeling of being out of control. The natural reaction, if not panic, is to want to seize control back. What became difficult for me and took many years to get over was the realization that I could not do so. Diabetes cannot be controlled. It's too overwhelming; it's too dangerous. But what I ultimately discovered was that my diabetes could be managed. You can't control a stormy sea, but you can manage the situation. You can ride it out and operate your boat with caution. So it is with diabetes. It was immensely empowering when I decided to surrender the idea of controlling my diabetes and determined instead to manage it.

Chronic conditions, in other words, are just like many aspects in our lives — all those things that you have to deal with on a day-to-day basis but that you can't necessarily control. Your boss, traffic, the weather, how well your favorite sports team is playing, etc. But in so far as they affect us, we can find ways to manage them, or plan around them, or react to them.

Reacting is the key because it all really adds up to this: if you can't change your situation, you can change your reaction to it. That's the one aspect you can control. We can't always control what happens to us in life, but we *can* choose how we're going to react. When it comes to your chronic condition, are you going to allow it to make you depressed, anxious, angry, fearful, or bitter? Or are you going to be happy and live your life as you wish to live it, notwithstanding whatever obstacles might be in your way? Everyone, it seems to me, chronic condition or not, without a doubt has this choice available to them every single day.

Choose happiness. Enjoy your life. Do the Snoopy dance.

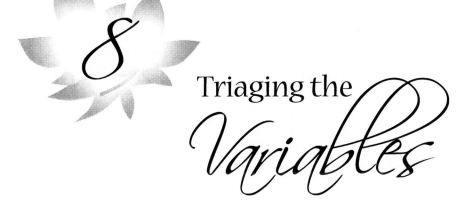

8

Triaging the *Variables*

"Chronic disease, like a troublesome relative, is something you can learn to manage but never quite escape. And while each and every person who has type 1 [diabetes] prays for a cure, and would give anything to stop thinking about it for just a year, a month, a week, a day even, the ironic truth is that only when you own it — accept it, embrace it, make it your own — do you start to be free of many of its emotional and physical burdens."

— Mary Tyler Moore

Managing diabetes, or celiac disease, or any chronic condition for that matter, starts with a very simple choice: deciding to want to manage it. Although that seems an obvious point, when a person is first diagnosed, the situation can often be too overwhelming for clearheaded thinking and determined actions. A chronic disease is scary enough in and of itself. But the task of learning how to manage it on a daily basis can be even more intimidating. When I was first diagnosed with diabetes, I remember being blasted with a fire hose of information that took me an extremely long time to sort out. And then of course there was that infuriating glucometer. There were many, many times when I just wanted to give up. Manage the disease? It seemed impossible.

Eventually, though, I simply reached a point where I realized that if I didn't properly manage my diabetes, my health and well-being were going to be severely jeopardized. My very life could be in danger. And I got tired of living with that kind of a cloud hovering over my head. I knew that — somehow — I was going to have to find a way to make my situation work. Life was going to go on, and I didn't want to let it pass me by. I wanted to enjoy my life and live it to the fullest. My desire to do so, in other words, ultimately trumped the fear I had that I wouldn't be able to properly manage my condition.

That didn't mean I could control it. In fact, what I discovered was that the idea of controlling such a monster was one of the things that was overwhelming me. But, as mentioned in the previous chapter, I knew that if I educated myself properly, I could manage it. I could make things work. I could live my life on my own terms. The diabetes would always be there, but I could find ways to work with it.

When I reached that point, I knew that I needed to somehow make use of that fire hose of information. Rather than allowing it to overwhelm me, I could take it in bits and pieces and learn from it. I might not have cared for how it was presented, but I also began to realize that, rather than being a discouraging, overpowering list of written-in-stone "can'ts" and "don'ts," the information was actually no more than a collection of recommendations and advice. Taken in that way, it didn't seem so overwhelming anymore. And I began to learn about managing my condition in a more open-minded way.

In time, my real education would come about from experience. I learned that serving sizes ("seventeen small grapes" or "one small banana") were not hard-and-fast rules. I began to understand more and more about what worked for me and what didn't. There was room for experimentation. Nothing drastic, mind you. But since every human body reacts differently than every other one, I knew that what would ultimately work for me couldn't possibly be simply pinned down to information published in some pamphlet.

Some of what I learned about my condition came the hard way. Shortly after I graduated from college, I went with a friend on a weekend backpacking trip. We hiked into the back country for a couple hours and set up camp. Everything was fine. But hiking back the next day, I found myself with serious blood sugar problems. I felt weak. Soon I began feeling exhausted, feeling as if I couldn't go on. My body wanted to rest but it seemed to me that if I stopped, if I sat down, I'd never make it back out. My blood sugar seemed unmanageable. With the help of my friend I kept myself going and we made it back to civilization, but it was a somewhat frightening ordeal. I'd learn later that my blood sugar had been bouncing around due to a phenomenon called rebounding. When my blood sugar was low, my body would produce glycogen as expected. But with diabetes, there's nothing to keep it in check. So my blood sugar would rise too high and I would take my insulin to bring it down, except that I ended up overcompensating with the insulin, resulting in a dangerous drop in blood sugar. Of course this caused even more production of glycogen and again dangerously high blood sugar which I overcompensated for again. The cycle of bouncing up and down continued. I wasn't aware of rebounding at the time. Not many people were, in fact. Rebounding was a fairly newly discovered phenomenon. But once I learned about it, I was able to take it into consideration, anticipate it, and plan around it. I might not be so quick to try to compensate for high blood sugar by giving myself extra insulin. You increase your knowledge with experience.

Actually, it's more than just experience. What's required is experience coupled with paying attention. Every time you find yourself with your blood sugar too low or too high, think of it as a learning opportunity. A single unacceptable glucometer reading might not tell you anything, but a few, at certain times, can help you spot patterns. Pay attention to the patterns. Make a note of them. There's no reason to panic about them (or want to smash The Machine into a million pieces), but rather you can learn from them. What's going on in your life during these patterns? What are you eating? What kind of physical activities are you engaging in? You become aware of your body and how it reacts to certain things when you just pay attention.

I know, for example, that in the winter months, I'm less active. And I've noticed over time that this affects my blood sugar. Knowing this allows me to properly compensate. Different foods (and at different times) also affect my blood sugar. Having some idea of the effect, I can try to minimize it. It's a process a friend of mind referred to as "triaging." When doctors triage patients, they prioritize them, making decisions based on all the available information at their disposal. I follow a similar strategy with my diabetes.

When it begins to feel overwhelming, which it routinely did for me especially after being diagnosed, I rely on a process that works towards smoothing out the ups and downs. Years after I began to use this process, I was pleasantly surprised to discover that the basic methodology behind it is what many successful corporations use to troubleshoot problems. Being something of a natural born troubleshooter, I guess it wasn't surprising that in my professional life I would gravitate to this very methodology; I became a certified Six Sigma Black Belt.

Six Sigma's philosophy is remarkably similar to the process I use to manage my diabetes: "reduce the variation, shift the mean." What this means is that if your blood sugar level is high over time, say 250 on average, work not to immediately reduce it to the optimal level, say, under 120, but rather seek to stabilize or even out your level (reduce the variation) and slowly bring the average down (shift the mean). Instead of swings from, for example, 75 to 300, reduce the extreme ups and downs by targeting readings ranging between 200 and 250. Once you are comfortable with your efforts, reset your target to 175 to 225. Then work on that range until you feel comfortable with your efforts and then aim for a new target. Reach your goal steadily, in a manageable, realistic, non-overwhelming way. Keep in mind that this is not an overnight process. It will take weeks or even months and it's important to be patient with yourself.

For me, the process involves striking a balance among four main variables: my eating, my stress level, my level of physical activity, and my insulin requirements. And it's ongoing. These variables are always in flux and always interacting with each other to produce new sets of conditions. Some of these conditions, based on experience, are more predictable than others. Even the more predictable ones, however, can surprise you.

If that seems frustrating, then welcome to life. Whether it's diabetes, a marriage, a career, or even just the weather, things are always changing. The key is to accept the changes and adapt to them. It's along the same idea as managing instead of controlling. We can choose to gather as much information as we can and make intelligent decisions about how to go forward. We can manage the situations we find ourselves in. We can triage our lives, in other words. Managing a chronic disease is not at all different from how we manage anything else.

Although I make every effort to achieve "normal" blood sugar levels, I know deep down that, for me, the goal of normal might not always be realistic. With a continual process, there's no single point you reach where you say, "There! I have now managed my condition perfectly." Understanding this is actually quite liberating. It's daunting and exhausting to go through life chained to a glucometer or HgA1c test, always afraid you won't measure up to the "perfect" standard the meter or test calls for. An imperfect reading or result is okay. Maybe I should have a blood sugar level of approximately 100 mg/dL. But if I'm at 130, or even 150, that's still okay. That's worth a small Snoopy dance. 200? Well, that might be a problem. I'll figure out why I'm there and make the appropriate correction. I'll triage. I'll get past it. If it's extremely low or high, I'd better triage quickly. That can be a more serious situation requiring immediate attention. But I'll get past that too. Better still, I'll learn from it. Whatever chain of events caused the high or low reading, I'll file it away in the back of my mind for future reference.

In this day and age of technology, it's easier to triage than when I was first diagnosed. Today, you can use a glucometer that allows you to download its data into a printable chart. You can easily spot patterns over time and make adjustments even more intelligently. This can be used along with your intuitive responses. After years of listening to your body, you become better able to trust your gut feeling. The Machine helps confirm your suspicions about what's going on with your blood sugar levels and, over time, you'll become more and more confident with your ability to manage, which will allow you to get on with your life.

9

Taming the *Sprue*

> *" The way to get started is to quit talking and begin doing. "*
>
> — Walt Disney

If diabetes can be challenging to manage, celiac disease can be just downright frustrating. At first glance it seems like it must be pretty easy — just avoid foods with gluten. Easier said than done. It's amazing the amount of foods that contain gluten, foods you would never suspect. A jar of nuts? Some brands actually use a light dusting of flour (wheat!) to keep the nuts from sticking together in the jar. Same with some brands of grated cheese. Blue cheese seems safe until you realize that it's made from mold — mold grown on … bread! Cross-contamination seems to be everywhere. When buying food at a grocery store, the secret is in diligently reading the labels. Same with medications. Yes, gluten can even show up in the drugstore, in both over-the-counter and prescription medications. Sometimes the "inactive" ingredients can be wheat-based. Read the label or ask your pharmacist or doctor.

Unfortunately, one cannot assume gluten isn't present. Recently, a friend of mine prepared chili for a get together, completely Gina-Friendly (Gluten-Free). Or so she thought. Upon further inspection, however, it turned out that the very first ingredient listed on the packet of seasoning she used was wheat flour. She felt awful when I told her I would prefer not to eat it. But I assured her that I sincerely appreciated her efforts and, besides, I was there for the camaraderie.

Restaurants provide their own sets of challenges. Of course I look for the G.F. designation. And although more and more restaurants are offering Gina-Friendly foods, they're still in the minority. That doesn't mean a restaurant won't have options that are Gina-Friendly. Sometimes you just have to ask. A lot of restaurants are familiar with the realities of gluten intolerance, even if their menus don't necessarily specify it. My rule of thumb is to ask, and then sort of govern my decision based on the reaction of the waiter or waitress. "Oh, yes, we have many gluten-free dishes available," is a very good sign. "Well … we have salads," followed by silence is, on the other hand, not such a good sign. Neither is: "Free what? Ma'am, we don't serve any free food here." And, yes, I've heard this more times than I like to think about.

Some restaurants cook their Gina-Friendly French fries in the same oil that they use to cook breaded foods, like onion rings. This kind of cross-contact means the fries come out not so Gina-Friendly. I always ask. Sometimes the server will jump right up and say, "Oh, yes, we use separate fryers." Other times I get a blank look and that tells me to stay away from the fries, if not the restaurant. If I question the food, I feel more confident when the server takes the initiative and tells me he or she will confirm with the chef. When someone just says, "Well, I'm pretty sure our grilled chicken is gluten-free," and then stands there waiting for my decision, I'm pretty sure I'm not going to order the chicken. In fact, I may never return to their restaurant.

Overall, I have found most restaurants are fairly understanding and accommodating. On a recent vacation with another couple, my husband and I stopped at a little place for lunch. After scouring the menu and talking to the waiter, I didn't feel very comfortable with the available choices. Looking out the window I spotted another restaurant across the street. We'd already ordered drinks and my husband and the other couple were satisfied with the place we were in. So, after they ordered, I simply asked the waiter if he would mind if I grabbed something from across the street and brought it back. "Not a problem at all," he assured me. I trotted across the street, ordered a gluten-free entrée to go, then came back and ate a nice lunch with the rest of my party.

Not everyone is comfortable asking for an accommodation like this. But in the management of any chronic condition, one has to be comfortable looking for work-arounds that might be a little outside of the box. You're simply going to have to make some concessions to the condition which might not always make things as convenient as you'd like them to be. But that doesn't mean you can't find ways to make things work.

The bottom line with the management of any chronic condition is to determine what works for you. Respect the disease. Understand the realities of the disease. But don't let it change who you are. Be *you*. And remember that it's always going to be a process. Learn from experience, adapt, and adjust.

10

Choosing Your Medical Support Team

The proper management of any chronic condition requires a little help. Support from your friends and family. Encouragement and advice, perhaps, from a support group or association. Maybe, most importantly, good medical treatment and guidance from your doctor or doctors.

The medical profession has come an amazingly long way in the treatment of chronic conditions such as diabetes. Prior to the discovery of insulin, less than a hundred years ago, a diagnosis of type 1 diabetes was essentially a death sentence. Insulin was lifesaving. Then came the ability for people to test their own blood sugar levels at home, rather than relying on testing one's urine, which often provided information that was, in reality, several hours old. Today, there are state-of-the-art glucometers. There is the HgA1c test, which reflects your blood glucose level over time, thus giving you a more accurate picture of how you're managing the disease in the long run. There are insulin pumps and insulin pens available. Tomorrow? Maybe a cure.

Medical science just keeps moving forward. If you have a chronic condition (or two), it often doesn't seem to. It frequently seems as though progress is being made at a snail's pace if any progress is being made at all. But after thirty-seven years of living with diabetes, I can look back and see the significant developments that have been made over that time. And in these days of information and technological advancement, changes can come out of nowhere. This is why it's important to keep on top of the latest information that's available about your chronic condition. And this is also why it's so important to take care of yourself today. You want your body to be in the best shape for any future advances, even cures. How tragic would it be if a cure came along but your health had, over time, become too badly deteriorated to take advantage of it?

With the Internet, keeping on top of the latest in medical advances is much easier today than it used to be. On the other hand, the amount of information you can find in a simple online search can be overwhelming. The information overload that results from any given query can stop you in your tracks. Where do you even start? How do you sort through it all? What's useful and what's not? What's really helpful and practical? What can even be trusted?

For me, I've found the best filter of the information onslaught is my own endocrinologist. More importantly, she knows how the latest information affects me specifically. Every patient is unique, with different needs and different responses to treatment.

What it comes down to is a relationship with my doctor that is collaborative. She's a trusted advisor, rendering valuable opinions and insights. If you don't feel as though you have this kind of connection with your doctor, you might want to consider finding another one. Not all doctors are alike. Just like there are no one-size-fits-all standards of treatment, there are no one-size-fits-all doctors.

I discovered this when I was first recommended to another endocrinologist by my primary care physician. This woman was a strict disciplinarian. When my blood sugar wasn't precisely where it needed to be, she let me know about it in no uncertain terms. She actually scolded me for my imperfection. She shook her head and said I was "not compliant." Ouch. That's a step away from "cheater." She never tried to find out what was happening, never asked me what I was or was not doing. She just made her blunt appraisal — I was not compliant — and that was that. I went back and told my primary care physician about my experiences and requested a referral to someone else. "But she's the best," he said. "Not for me," I said.

That particular endocrinologist was quite a contrast from my very first endocrinologist, now retired. Dr. Robert Beshore was the doctor who gave me that understanding look back when I had said that one day I slept in past the time to take my insulin because I just wanted to feel normal. He seemed to get me, he seemed to appreciate my feelings about my condition, my fears and concerns. Far from a disciplinarian, he was more of a partner. I learned from him, and he learned from me as well. He learned from all his patients. Once when he was considering whether or not to recommend a new insulin pump for his patients, he felt that the best way to find out was to try it himself. And so he wore one, filled with a simple saline solution, for a couple days, just so he could let his patients know honestly how the pump worked and what it felt like. That's the kind of doctor I can appreciate. And I actually used one of those pumps for several years, making me one of the first to do so. The pumps back then were about the size of your average small paperback. Of course now they're about as small as a cell phone.

Once, during a bout of insecurity, when I was certain an HgA1c test would show that I wasn't managing my diabetes properly, Dr. Beshore, who had more faith in me than I had, assured me it would instead show that I was just fine. "Wanna bet?" I asked. "Sure," he replied. We bet a Diet Coke. I was sure the result would be over 8 (high). He was sure it would be under 8, maybe 7.4. It was 7.5. I thanked him for his encouragement and on my way out of his office, stopped off at a vending machine. Then I ducked back into his office and set a can of Diet Coke on his desk. He smiled. So did I. It was a bet I was happy to lose.

I enjoy a similar relationship with my current endocrinologist too. Although it's the doctor's goal to get your blood sugar levels as close to normal as possible — like that of a nondiabetic person — it's not always going to happen and it is not always easy. What I have with my endocrinologist today is someone who understands that I will try — always — to do my best. But sometimes I'm going to come up a little short. At these times, I don't need a lecture and a scolding and to be told I am not compliant. I need to be able to sit down with my doctor and talk about ways to improve my situation. I need advice, advice that will work for me and will work, especially, for my lifestyle.

This idea of collaboration is important to me. I consulted with a dietitian once, wanting a better understanding of my dietary needs and restrictions and maybe some creative ideas and more flexible options. The dietitian was someone I was referred to and she listened to all my concerns (at least I think she was listening) but then promptly handed me a pamphlet with all the dos and don'ts. I said thanks and left her office and never went back. I can go online and find what she provided me in about two minutes and not even have to leave the house. On the other hand, I asked a doctor one time about replenishing fluids after working out. I was concerned about a particular juice beverage I'd been drinking. He thought for a second and said, "Dilute it 60/40 with water, Gina. And that should be fine." It was simple advice but it was constructive and educated. And it took into account my particular circumstance. It was the kind of information you probably won't find on a pamphlet. It was advice that was appropriate *for the context* of the situation. That's the kind of collaborative relationship I'm looking for in a doctor.

This is not to discount the value of firm guidelines and credible lists of what one should eat or drink and the respective serving sizes. I know some people living with diabetes who prefer strict rules. And they also need a doctor who's more of a disciplinarian. They respond well to the idea that if they're not doing the appropriate job in managing their disease, they're going to get an earful from their doctor. Without that underlying threat, they may become lax. It really comes down to what type of person you want, and need, on your team. Overall, you need to feel comfortable that you have the right doctor for you, one that relates to you and one to whom you can relate.

Whether you feel as though you need strict rules or not, there are some people who feel as if every doctor is a disciplinarian. Anyone with a white coat and stethoscope makes them anxious. In truth, we all feel this a little bit. It's test anxiety. Sometimes going to the doctor makes us feel the same way we might feel going in to take that big final exam we've been studying for. Will we pass? Will the doctor tell us everything is all right? Or will he or she look at our chart and give us that serious furrowed brow (I think they learn that in med school) and say something like, "Hmm … I'm not sure I like this." Test anxiety? Maybe it's more like being sent to the principal's office.

It's a common feeling. Interestingly enough, my endocrinologist admitted to having the feeling when she goes to her own doctor! No wonder so many people avoid the doctor or delay office visits. For some people with chronic conditions, a visit to the doctor is a reminder of their chronic condition, something they'd rather not have to think about. But it's necessary, and if you have the appropriate doctor in place for you, then you can at least feel a level of comfort. You're not always going to feel happy going to the doctor's office, but you should at least feel comfortable. You should at least feel as though you're in the right hands.

My appointments with my endocrinologist, or primary care physician for that matter, are, to my way of thinking, consultative meetings. My doctor has her agenda, but I also have mine. It's not uncommon for me to come into the examination room with a written list of questions I've been saving up. Maybe there's a new treatment I read about in a magazine or on the Internet. Maybe something unexpected happened with my blood sugar level recently for which I hope to get an explanation, or educated opinion, at least. The doctor is my counsel. Always remember that it's your health at stake. Don't be afraid to ask questions. And if you don't understand the answers, keep asking.

Ultimately, of course, you have to be responsible for your own health. Your doctor or doctors can only do so much. But my experience has shown me that a doctor is more willing to work with you if the doctor knows that you are doing your best to take your condition seriously. My first endocrinologist suggested the insulin pump to me precisely because he knew that

I would be diligent with it and use it properly. He knew I was a responsible patient. And he also knew that I was willing to try new treatment options in the hopes of being able to better manage my diabetes.

If you're serious about facing your condition, you'll find you don't have to face it all alone. Medical science can help and with the right team in place, with the right people overseeing your health, you can not only feel safer and more secure, you can thrive. Seek out the right doctor for you and take charge of your health by taking advantage of all the help, guidance, and latest developments the medical community has to offer.

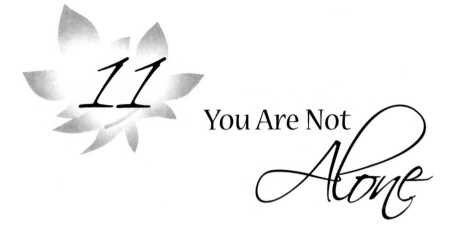

11

You Are Not *Alone*

> *Lots of people want to ride with you in the limo, but what you want is someone who will take the bus with you when the limo breaks down.*
>
> — Oprah Winfrey

In addition to your medical team there are other sources of ongoing support as well, some of which might help you not just physically but emotionally. For your particular chronic condition, there are no doubt organized support groups available right where you live. A lot of times these groups can provide a forum where you can ask questions or maybe just express your frustrations, a welcome place where there are others who understand what you're feeling.

The best groups, however, are those that have real, valuable information to share. Yes, it's sometimes important — especially early on in one's experience with a chronic disease where, perhaps, the struggle to accept it is still playing out — to have a place where you can commiserate with others and be offered some sympathy. But if that ends up being the only real focus of the support group, it can become a place where people go just to wallow. That doesn't help anyone — not the people who are expressing their frustration by grumbling about their condition, nor those who are sitting there listening to the grumbling. A chronic condition is difficult. Everyone knows that. There's only so much that can be said about that part of it and after a while, the grumbling all starts to sound the same. Better, I think, to find a group whose attitude seems to primarily reflect thinking that is positive, a group that shares helpful ideas, tips, and valuable, practical advice.

For four years, I served as president of such a group: the Denver Metro Chapter of the Celiac Sprue Association (CSA), a national organization committed to helping those with gluten intolerance through education, awareness, and research. I originally joined to learn as much as I could about celiac disease. I wanted some helpful ideas about what kind of food I should look for and where I could find it. For the most part that's what I found. But I noticed there was still a certain level of grumbling that went on, sometimes even wallowing. As president, I tried to redirect the grumbling into something positive. At one meeting a member was lamenting the lack of gluten-free beer choices, especially in restaurants and bars. He went on for several minutes about it, until I finally suggested that there might be ways to work around the problem. I related my experience of meeting some friends at a local bar on a beautiful summer afternoon. The bar had an outdoor patio and I wanted nothing more than to sit outside with my friends and share a beer with them. But the bar didn't have any beer that was gluten-free. I explained my situation to the manager and he was willing to allow me to carry out to the patio a gluten-free brand of beer that I had brought with me. I had to be discreet, of course; customers bringing their own beers into the bar wasn't exactly a precedent he wanted to publicize. I stuck a beer in my purse and headed outside to sit with my friends. Maybe that won't work everywhere, but that wasn't the point. I just wanted to let him know that if you think outside the box, sometimes you can work around a problem. What I left unsaid — but think he understood — is that sitting around bemoaning all of the possible obstacles, instead of looking for potential solutions, isn't very helpful.

I always tried to foster a positive can-do atmosphere in our chapter meetings, to make it a place where people were optimistic and encouraging. Collectively, we looked for solutions to problems and ways in which to make life a lot easier. I'm proud to be the founder of a gluten-free food fair, for example, inviting restaurants and food vendors to bring samples of their products. It was a way for them to introduce their gluten-free foods to a receptive audience and it went over fairly well. Twenty vendors came and about 200 people attended in the inaugural year. Now, six years later, the "Incredible, Edible Gluten-Free Food Fair™" — as we call it — brings in close to a hundred vendors and over 3,000 attendees. That's the kind of creative thinking that a good support group ought to try to foster. It's the kind of thing that you, too, ought to try to foster; all it takes is some imagination and a determination to look for solutions instead of problems.

If you're living with gluten intolerance, check out your local chapter of the Celiac Sprue Association. You can go to their main website at www.csaceliacs.info. Another valuable organization is the Gluten Intolerance Group (GIG). Check them out at www.gluten.net. For diabetes, the trusted authority is the American Diabetes Association (ADA) at www.diabetes.org.

These organizations, and others like them, can be extremely helpful in providing you with ongoing support.

In addition to your doctors, family, and friends, and whatever support groups you may choose to affiliate yourself with, your chief source of support might be your significant other. This may especially be true on an emotional level. A chronic condition can test to the limit the "through sickness and health" part of the marriage vows. But I have found over the course of a twenty-four-year marriage that with love, respect, and good communication, a chronic condition needn't test a marriage any more than the myriad other things that are inherent in any long-term committed relationship. The keys are openness, honesty, and a willingness to share.

It also helps to know what you're getting into. When I first met my husband Jim, I had already been diagnosed with diabetes. Jim knew about my condition right from the start and for him, it was, as he puts it, "just part of the package." I was wearing an insulin pump at the time and Jim will tell you that his only real concern was that he had to be careful touching me and putting his arms around me for fear of knocking the pump loose or bumping up against the point of injection.

His patience was tested a little more than that, though, during one particular Christmas early on in our relationship. I ended up in the hospital on Christmas Day, suffering from the effects of the flu and having an extremely difficult time managing my blood sugar. It happens. But my experience as a young adult, having to be airlifted to the hospital in a coma, had made me wiser. Jim got a real close look at the challenges a person living with diabetes sometimes has to face. I remember him telling me that one of my family members made the remark that the hospital visit was something of a blessing. "Now Jim can see what he's really getting into," they said. To which Jim's sister Janet had this to say: "Yes, and now Gina can see what kind of man Jim really is."

If you're not going to get the support you need from your significant other, where are you going to get it? It's all a part of the commitment you make to each other. Jim was reminded of this once again about six months after our wedding day. This time it was an intestinal problem that didn't even have anything to do with my diabetes. But it was an emergency situation and Jim had to race me to the hospital after coming home to find me doubled over in pain. I ended up needing abdominal surgery and while I was recovering, my father put it all into perspective for Jim. Tired, and wanting to take a break from the hospital waiting room, they decided to go out for coffee. Sitting in a coffee shop, my father, in his strong Irish brogue, turned to Jim with a long and serious face.

"Well, laddie," he began, "I've got to tell you something."

"What's that?" Jim replied apprehensively, not knowing at all where the conversation with my father was suddenly headed.

Said my father: "The warranty's up, I'm afraid. And now she's all yours."

They both had a well-needed laugh.

With my celiac diagnosis, it was a little different. Jim could accept the diabetes as part of the Gina package without necessarily having to make any really significant day-to-day adjustments to his own life. For celiac, he had to learn, along with me, the many things one needs to know to avoid potential problems. The smallest details need to always be considered. Using a knife, for example, to spread peanut butter on a piece of bread and then putting the knife back into the peanut butter jar can cause cross-contamination. Becoming, and remaining, aware of all of the possible hazards required lifestyle modifications not just for me, but for Jim as well. Today, he's a diligent label-reader and he's on constant guard for potential sources of gluten that might be lurking around.

It's not always easy for him, but it's given him a chance to help, to do something to make a difference. "Men," Jim likes to say, "are natural problem solvers and hunter-gatherers." With my diabetes, he often helps with gentle reminders, encouraging me sometimes to check my blood sugar, especially at times when I might not want to bother, times that I'm sick, for instance. With my celiac disease, he can take even more positive action. He can search out foods and beverages and restaurants, and do helpful research.

Jim's careful, though, not to try to take over. Assisting someone with a chronic condition is one thing. Attempts to control it or manage it, though carried out perhaps with the best of intentions, is something else. A person with a chronic condition needs to be able to manage it on their own. The person affected has to take charge of the condition him or herself. It might be tempting to want to do everything for a loved one who has diabetes or celiac disease, but the person living with diabetes or celiac needs the freedom to overcome, by way of their own efforts, the inherent difficulties of their condition or conditions. This is where real growth comes from. Having everything done for you, even if it's out of love, is a form of enabling and what might seem helpful ends up being stifling.

Ultimately, the support you receive from your spouse ought to depend on what kind of support you need. This is different for everybody. Some people need more emotional support. Some people need more practical day-to-day help. No matter what your support requirements are, don't assume they're obvious to your significant other. And if you're the significant other, don't just assume you know what your partner needs. Both parties need to communicate. Ask questions. Listen. Jim will tell you this is by far the most important factor in living — as a couple — with a chronic condition.

For my part, just knowing Jim is going to be there for me is the best support. He accepted the diabetes as "part of the package." With the diagnosis of celiac disease, he had to accept something else about me. But he made it clear from the start that we were going to handle it together. I was not going to be alone. But then again, as Jim likes to remind me, what else could he do? "I couldn't very well take you back," he says. "After all, your warranty was up."

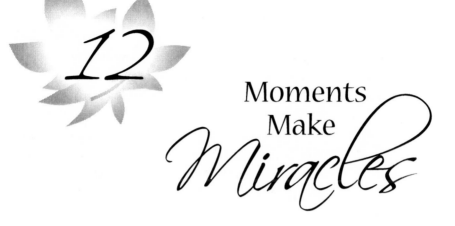

12
Moments
Make
Miracles

In discussing this book with my niece, I mentioned that my purpose for writing was not to try to declare that chronic conditions like diabetes or celiac disease are somehow easy to live with. They most certainly are not. Amanda happens to also be living with celiac disease, so she knows. But, as I explained to her, I just wanted to give people a different way to perhaps think of their situation. And then Amanda reminded me of the way I had put it to her: "You have to think of your disease," she said, "not as a hindrance, but as a lifestyle change."

If there's a quick way to sum it all up, that's it. There are, after all, as many different lifestyles as lives, it seems to me. Everyone has his or her own way of living, his or her own problems and difficulties to live with and manage, his or her own burdens to carry. If you've just been diagnosed with a chronic condition, you now have a different set of circumstances in your life to deal with. But with time and patience and the right mindset, you can find ways to not only deal with your new circumstances — your new lifestyle — but to flourish.

Patience might be the key. Remember that properly and effectively managing your condition is not something that typically happens overnight. It might take years before you feel comfortable with how you're managing things. Even today, I know that my diabetes can present a problem at any time. I might be perfectly fine one day and in the hospital the next. But I also know that's a rare occurrence, made even more rare over time simply by my experience in managing my diabetes. Still, the concern is real. I have to — always — take my condition seriously. While at the same time, living my life as I want to live it. That's the balance that must be struck. I got there. And you can get there too.

Remember, though, that life is a journey and not a destination. Every day is new and every day brings fresh challenges. Every day also brings fresh opportunities and new learning experiences. Living with a chronic condition — more precisely, perhaps, learning to live with a chronic condition (or two) — is an ongoing process. Even after all this time, I still have days that are hard, emotionally, if not physically. And I always will, because there's no finish line but one and God willing, that's a long ways off. Until then, each day has to be considered in its own right; life starts anew every morning.

One thing that helps my attitude is that I allow myself permission to fail. I'm going to try, for example, to always keep my blood sugar where it ought to be. But I also know that some-times, despite my best efforts, I'm going to miss the mark. That machine, cold and impersonal, will call me out on it and tell me I've failed. But that's okay. What The Machine doesn't know is that any particular reading is just a single moment in time, a point on a long continuum. Once I came to understand that, I stopped being afraid of The Machine. It tells me when I might need to make an adjustment, and it tells me when I've done well. That's all. And when I've done well, I celebrate. I do the Snoopy dance. Find a way to celebrate *your* successes. You deserve it!

Remember that you are much, much more than the chronic condition you are living with. One thing that I've never done, and refuse to do, is call myself "a diabetic." Or a "victim" of celi-ac disease. I'm a person living with diabetes. I'm a person living with celiac disease. My conditions do not define me. They are part of me, but they are not who I am or what I am all about. Don't let your conditions define you, either.

I don't allow myself to be defined by other negative terms, either. If I eat a piece of chocolate, I am not a "cheater." I don't cheat. I am not "noncompliant." Words have meanings and terms like these, repeated over and over again, will seep into your very psyche and affect your mindset, even your sense of self-worth. What I learned over time is that, within reason, I can do whatev-er I want. I have choices. I assumed when I was diagnosed with diabetes that my freedom of choice had been taken away. Not so. I fully understand, however, that there might be consequences to my choices and I factor those into my decision-making pro-cess. But whatever I do, the choice is mine and whatever choice I make, I am most certainly *not* cheating.

Along those lines, I have come to understand that the lists of dos and don'ts that are provided to people with chronic conditions are *guidelines* only. Seventeen small grapes? A less-than-six-inch banana? Everyone is different. The lists represent rough ballpark estimates at best. If you like the specificity of the lists, if the structure is important to you, then by all means follow the lists. But understand that doing so is still a choice. You have the power to decide whether you're going to eat seventeen small grapes as recommended, or twenty, or none.

Making choices, smart choices, is all a part of the bigger picture of properly managing your condition — managing it physically as well as managing it emotionally. And managing is the best you'll be able to do. There is no "controlling" of your disease. Part of the acceptance process is understanding this. It's natural to want to think you can control your disease and ultimately be its master. But eventually you realize how exhausting this way of thinking is. It becomes intimidating and frustrating and hopelessly discouraging. When you decide to let go of the idea of controlling and instead focus on managing, life becomes a *lot* easier. Managing is realistic. Managing is something you can accomplish today.

In the end, I've learned that living with a chronic condition is best approached in the exact same way in which anyone needs to approach their life, with or without a chronic condition: one day at a time. By focusing on what's before you today, you can make this day special. Tomorrow, you can do the same thing. Put a few days together and you've got a week and the weeks roll into months and the next thing you know, you're not living with a chronic condition, you're *flourishing*. I know from experience. I know what's available to you. Life awaits you, with all of its wonders. All you have to do is decide that, just for today, nothing's going to stop you.

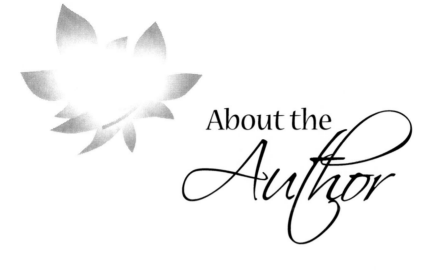

About the *Author*

Gina Meagher was diagnosed with type 1 diabetes at the age of seventeen. At thirty-two, she was diagnosed with celiac disease. Understandably, both chronic conditions have been challenging and frustrating for her. But they've also been educational and, over time, Gina has learned not only how to live with the conditions, but how to flourish in spite of them. *There Is Something about Gina* is the result of her desire to share her experiences and insights for the benefit of others who may be struggling with diabetes, celiac, or other chronic conditions. Gina has a unique perspective that is supportive and encouraging, practical and helpful. Former president of the Denver Metro Chapter of the Celiac Sprue Association, and founder of the Denver Chapter of the Incredible, Edible Gluten-Free Food Fair™, Gina is a frequent speaker on the subject of living with chronic conditions. She currently resides in Golden, Colorado, with her husband Jim.

CPSIA information can be obtained
at www.ICGtesting.com
Printed in the USA
LVOW11s1329180618
581083LV00001B/81/P